EVERYTHING

YOU NEED TO KNOW ABOUT...

Organizing
Your home

EVERYTHING

YOU NEED TO KNOW ABOUT...

Organizing Your Home

Jenny Schroedel

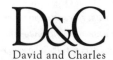
David and Charles

This book is dedicated to my mom, masterful organizer and skillful homemaker,
for creating a home that I'm always eager to get back to.

A DAVID & CHARLES BOOK
Updates and amendments copyright © David & Charles Limited 2007
Copyright © 2007 F+W Publications Inc.
Front cover image © Lakeland Ltd

David & Charles is an F+W Publications Inc. company
4700 East Galbraith Road
Cincinnati, OH 45236

First published in the UK in 2007
First published in the USA as The Everything® Organizing Your Home Book,
by Adams Media in 2007

A catalogue record for this book is available from the British Library.

ISBN-13: 978-0-7153-2838-5
ISBN-10: 0-7153-2838-7

Printed in Great Britain by Antony Rowe Ltd
for David & Charles
Brunel House, Newton Abbot, Devon

Visit our website at www.davidandcharles.co.uk

David & Charles books are available from all good bookshops;
alternatively you can contact our Orderline on 0870 9908222 or
write to us at FREEPOST EX2 110, D&C Direct, Newton Abbot,
TQ12 4ZZ (no stamp required UK only).

Contents

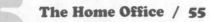

Acknowledgments

I wish to gratefully acknowledge the tireless efforts of my editor, Kerry Smith, for her prompt and thorough responses to my questions and for her encouraging tone throughout this project. I also want to thank my mom for reading chapters and offering helpful suggestions, as well as my husband, John, and daughter, Anna, for bearing with me as I tackled this book, and for working with me as we seek to bring order to our home.

Top Ten Organizational Commandments

1. **Know yourself.** Before organizing, identify psychological blocks, problems with your technique, and your organizational goals. This knowledge will help you toward long-term success.

2. **Be flexible.** Different phases of life—a new marriage, a new child, divorce, or a death in the family—present organizational challenges. Modify your systems and give yourself time to integrate these changes.

3. **Be kind to yourself.** In most cases, organizational challenges have nothing to do with laziness or incompetence. Other root causes are at the heart of your struggle. This book will help you to identify them.

4. **Be gentle with others.** As you become organizationally zealous, your family might irritate you. Work toward reasonable compromises.

5. **Enlist the crew.** Don't purge others' belongings when they're not around. Instead, develop systems that work for everyone.

6. **Banish perfection.** Your home is occupied by living beings with mess-making capacities. Home organization, especially for those with little ones, is always a work in progress.

7. **Watch your wallet.** Before you max out your credit cards, develop a plan.

8. **Combat clutter.** Keep excess out of your home. When you acquire something new, let go of something old. Only keep items that are beautiful, are useful, or have significant emotional value.

9. **Make it fun.** As you organize, pipe in music or a radio program you love and be sure to reward yourself for each success along the way.

10. **Love your home.** Even if you don't live in the home of your dreams, relish the elements of your dwelling that bring you joy.

Introduction

▶ IF YOU'VE PICKED UP THIS BOOK, you're probably itching to get organized. Maybe your house is in pretty good shape, but the garage and attic are completely out of control. Or perhaps your home is so chaotic that you have to dig a trail through the clutter to get from your front door to your kitchen. Whatever your situation is, this book can help you as you take small, concrete steps toward your goals.

The struggle for order is always against the backdrop of the rush to get the kids to school on time, pay the bills, manage challenges at work and at home, and get the oil changed. Henry David Thoreau wrote, "Our life is frittered away by detail." Sometimes you might feel so busy just managing the details of life that domestic goals—such as clearing out your garage so you can park there this winter—can go ignored for months (or years) at a time.

This book is for all of us who struggle to balance all those details, yet stubbornly persist in our desire for an orderly home. The tips in this book are intended for those who have just a few minutes a day (and perhaps a few hours a day over the weekend) to organize. As you work through the chapters in this book, take the advice that will work for your own situation, and leave the rest. Feel free to skip around and read the chapters that intrigue you or are most directly related to your current organizational challenges. You can keep the book for reference as new challenges present themselves over the years.

The most important thing is that you find an approach that works for you. Perhaps you've purchased organizational books in the past, latched on to a particular method with enthusiasm, and wrestled your home (and life) into order, only to have the mess return a few months later. This book will help you develop a customized approach to your own unique, internalized organizational challenges. If you can develop an approach that fits your personality and circumstance, you're far more likely to be able to achieve long-term success.

This book explores some of the psychological blocks on the path to organization, and it also offers a huge variety of organizational tips and strategies. Room by room, you'll have an opportunity to explore ways to sort, purge, and organize your belongings. But this book isn't just about organizing—it is also about creating a home that you'll love to come back to.

Organizing is a significant piece of the equation, but it is not everything. It is equally important to develop cleaning strategies that are efficient, realistic, and—in some cases—fun. If you've attempted in the past to bring order to your home, then you're well aware of the other hidden struggle behind the chaos—life with other people. This book will also offer practical tools for navigating the emotional landmines that are often hidden in those thickets of clutter.

Homes are not unlike living beings—they need to breathe, they need to be nurtured and loved, and they have a profound relationship with the emotional, spiritual, and financial dimensions of life. As you come to better understand the obstacles that are holding you back, as well as the opportunities that await you, you'll be better able to chart a course through the clutter and to find ways to bring about long-term change.

Although organizing is never effortless, it doesn't have to be a chore. As you tackle the chaos in your home one drawer at a time, you'll find that the work has its own rewards. It often feels so good to sort and purge that ,over time, you might get hooked on the process. The joy you find in this work, as well as your increasing ability to experience the beauty of your home, will help you to persist in your efforts and to create a place that you'll love coming home to day after day.

Chapter 1

Time to Kick the Clutter Habit

The first step in organizing your home is to purge. Too much clutter will make the task overwhelming and oppressive. Once you've managed to clear out a bit of the excess, you'll be better able to prioritize and to feel that you are capable of tackling the tasks at hand. This chapter will explore the emotional dimensions of clutter—the interpersonal struggles surrounding it, as well as the fresh possibilities that a streamlined home create.

When Clutter Suffocates

Homes all over America are brimming with clutter. Closets are stuffed to capacity, triggering a small avalanche each time one is opened, every flat surface is piled with paper, and the basement and attic are filled with unidentifiable items. This kind of situation can obscure even the most beautiful homes.

Ideally, a home is an oasis of peace, rest, and comfort in the midst of a chaotic world. But keeping out the chaos is no small undertaking. The mailbox brims with junk mail and catalogs, and products in every mall cry out, "Take me home!" Each holiday brings a fresh deluge from well-meaning friends and family.

When clutter begins to take over, it can become almost impossible to find solace in a home. Instead of feeling a wave of peace rush over you when you pass through the door, you might instead feel a sense of dread, duty, or guilt. You might hope to get to it all one day, but the task only seems to grow more daunting with time. The temptation is to just put it off indefinitely. You might say to yourself, "I'll try to do that tomorrow, or when the kids are back in school . . . or maybe when they head off to college."

This temptation, while it might be enticing, is really only a means of prolonging the agony. And it is draining to live in a home that continually drags you down, demanding more from you than you are able to give it.

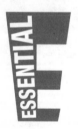

How does clutter makes you feel? Try to be aware of your emotional response to overstuffed closets and chaotic drawers. Do you feel helpless, depressed, or angry? Realize that although those emotions are part of life, you do have the power to begin to take small steps toward transforming your environment, as well as the emotions that environment evokes.

Clutter steals space from the more precious things in life, complicating daily rituals and intensifying already stressful situations. Have you ever tried to track down a lone shoe in an abyss of a closet for a preschooler who is already late for school? Ever been tardy to a meeting because you were searching for an important document in mountains of paper? Ever miss a credit card payment because the bill got caught in a stack of unread newspapers?

When the home is cluttered, simple things in life become complicated. Life can feel as frenzied and chaotic as our homes. Clutter consumes time, energy, and psychic space that could be spent enjoying your children, cooking a nice meal, or sipping coffee on the window seat and watching the world go by.

When clutter suffocates, it not only steals time, it saps energy. If you find that you are consistently exhausted in your own home, it might be clutter that is dragging you down. There is a physical component to this emotional experience—piles of paper, books, and clothing attract dust mites and other allergens. Not only does it feel harder to breathe in a cluttered home, it *is* harder to breathe!

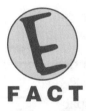

FACT

According to the principles of feng shui, cluttered corners trap precious energy and restrict the flow of life through homes. Ideally, clutter will be purged out of your home so that energy can move freely through the home. This practice could result in a much more restful home environment for you and your family.

The FlyLady, Marla Cilley (*www.flylady.net*), the founder of the SHE (Sidetracked Home Executive) organizational method, has helped countless families get their homes in order through her writing, her Web site, her Yahoo group, and her e-mail list. She refers to the areas of our homes that consistently attract clutter as "hot zones," because while they can be easy to ignore, they demand our attention. When ignored, they grow, stealing more and more space from our homes, like weeds that are ignored for too long and slowly begin to choke the life out of the tomato plants, snapdragons, and lilies in the garden.

Room to Breathe

After you've considered how clutter makes you feel, and if the feelings produced are largely negative, know that these emotions are a red flag urging you to explore a new way of thinking about and living in your home. Perhaps it is impossible to imagine this now, but almost as easily as clutter comes into your home, you can get it out.

By packing up the clutter and removing it from your home, you begin to reclaim your space and your time. Although this task requires effort—and demands some measure of consistency—it also gives something back. By eliminating excess from your life, you create space to breathe.

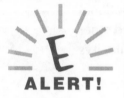

Clutter often takes years to accumulate, and it will take time to remove it all. Beware of perfectionist thinking—you do not need to tackle every closet in one afternoon. Instead, begin to break projects into steps, and try to devote a small segment of time to this work each day.

In an uncluttered home, you can see more clearly. If you clear your dining room table, for example, and polish it to a shine, you might be surprised at how beautiful it is. If you make your bed each day and reserve that space for sleep and comfort, you might find it easier to drift off each night. And if you can keep your desk reasonably clear and tidy, you communicate to yourself that you are a productive person, ready to face the tasks at hand, and capable of managing them, one job at a time.

Most of all, by clearing the clutter out of your home, you create space— space to rest, space to comfort, space to love. The FlyLady calls the every-day work of ordering a home a "house blessing," because you are literally blessing your home with your actions, bringing order out of chaos and beauty out of ugliness.

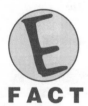

According to professional organizer Julie Morgenstern, a fear of success might sometimes be at the heart of chaos. As long as the clutter and chaos remain, one is always distracted and never able to fully focus on their aspirations. This kind of mess can also convey to the world (and to oneself) that a person is not worthy of success.

When you "bless" your home on a regular basis, you are less likely to feel as if you need to go elsewhere for rest and relaxation. Instead, the home becomes the center of comfort and you can draw strength from it. Instead of fancy meals and retail therapy, you might find that your own home has everything you need to feel sane, settled, and content.

The Childhood Roots of Adult Clutter

The tendency to hoard objects is often passed from one generation to the next. Clutter is never just about "stuff." Your possessions represent essential links to other people, and to ideas you have about yourself. Most people are pretty oblivious about the messages they unconsciously received as children that continue to influence their actions today.

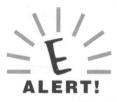

Clutter can have a negative effect on your social life, especially if the fear of letting others see your home keeps you from entertaining. As you begin to bring order to your home, your confidence will grow and you might be able to widen your circle of friends as well.

For those who experienced trauma as children—such as the death of a parent, a divorce, or extreme poverty—material possessions may be loaded with far more meaning than their mere physical value. A person might be tempted to hold on to items they no longer need because at some point in their lives, they lost something (or someone) they deeply valued. The pain of this loss may cause them to think that the only way they can protect themselves from more loss is to accumulate things. The stuff they accumulate becomes an armor of sorts, creating a kind of insulation from the ravages of the outside world, but also keeping a person trapped inside.

What's Divorce Got to Do with It?

In the book *Between Two Worlds: The Inner Lives of Children of Divorce,* Elizabeth Marquardt interviews numerous adult children of divorce to see how their childhood experiences impact their lives today. One of the chapters is entirely devoted to questions surrounding "stuff." For many adult children of divorce, the experience of having their parents separate meant more than a change in family structure. It may have caused a move from a large house to a two-bedroom apartment. It may have meant that quickly, without warning and under extreme pressure, these children had to give up multiple items that they treasured. This kind of experience can cause a person to believe that no matter how much stuff they have, they need to hold on to it all, because they never know what change is around the bend.

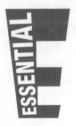

If you find yourself holding on to items long after they've outlived their use (for purely emotional reasons), consider taking a photo of the object to be stored in your digital files. That way, you retain a record of the person or experience associated with the object, without retaining the burden of the object itself.

Just as trauma can sometimes be passed from one generation to the next—as can tendencies toward alcoholism, emotional or physical abuse, or mental illness—the tendency to hoard material objects can easily pass from one generation to the next. If your parents (unconsciously) taught you that hoarding was necessary, they may have also conveyed to you that no matter how many possessions you owned, you would never have enough. These kinds of messages can be a huge stumbling block to a person who hopes to live in an orderly, serene, and uncluttered environment.

The Need for Abundance

The first step on the path to overcoming these messages is to learn what they are. So often, people, especially children, receive messages uncritically. From your adult perspective, try to think about what your parents conveyed to you through their relationship with stuff. If they had a deprivation mentality, you might also feel a great need for abundance.

In Julie Morgenstern's book *Organizing from the Inside Out*, she writes about a deep-seated need that many people have for abundance. It is her theory that these are the people who consistently buy in bulk and struggle to let go of things even when they are no longer useful.

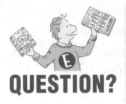

QUESTION?

Does having clutter around make it more difficult for me to clean my house?
Yes! Professional cleaners estimate that by eliminating clutter, cleaning time can be reduced by as much as 40 percent.

Morgenstern does not believe that pack rats must become purgers. Instead, she feels that it is most ideal to work with a person's need for abundance instead of trying to thwart it. In contrast to most philosophies of home organizing, she does not demand that her clients immediately purge. Instead, she tries to help them bring order to their environment, and expects that as the order improves, people become more discerning about their possessions.

In contemporary consumer culture, it is often far easier to acquire things than it is to purge them. If your parents hoarded multiple useless items because they "might need them someday," you might have inherited a similar attitude toward possessions. To be fair, there are many purgers out there who do manage to get rid of possessions they still need and may be forced to go out to the store to replace items that they once owned. Blind zeal can be as dangerous for the purger as it is for the pack rat.

Still, it is often easier to replace certain items when necessary than it is to manage multiple unused items in your home. Keep this in mind if you want a clean, orderly home—clutter resists clean. The first critical battle for the home organizer is the war on clutter. If you can begin to develop a strategic approach to clutter, you'll be in a much better position to bring order to your home.

While people may disagree about how streamlined a home needs to be, it is clear that finding ways to simplify your life does help with organization. As Victoria Moran wrote in her book *Shelter for the Spirit*, "Be forewarned: If you organize before you simplify, things will be disorganized again in no time. This is not because you're a hopeless slob without a prayer for redemption. It is because excess cannot be organized. If it could, it would not be excess."

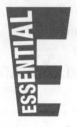

What kind of relationship did your parents have with material possessions? How does their attitude toward material objects influence the way you see these things today? Take a moment and write down some of the messages that they consciously (or unconsciously) conveyed to you.

After you've begun to put words to the messages that influence the way you manage your possessions, you'll be in a better position to begin to change. Self-awareness is the key to transformation in every area of life. Before you can change how you are, you must first understand how you became that way and what hidden factors might be behind your actions. As you begin to know yourself better (and identify the messages that have influenced you for years), you might find that you are in a better position to begin to combat clutter. Now, instead of just blindly living by these messages, you can begin to let go of those messages that weren't helpful, while still holding on to the ones that were.

Living with Others

The daily grind of life with another person can be exhausting. It can be daunting to come up against another person's will and desires, to realize that your own plans and ideas may need to be revised on a regular basis to accommodate the other person. The daily work of compromise and negotiation requires no small effort, even for those in happy families.

This struggle certainly extends to the home, where, in almost every relationship, each person has a different idea about clutter. For one person, a semi-cluttered space is conducive to comfort and productivity. For another, a stripped-down, sparse environment is necessary. Mike Mason, the author of *The Mystery of Marriage*, writes candidly of the "bitter and ironic truth that the very person we love most in the world may appear to us, from time to time, to be the only thing standing between ourselves and our happiness."

Likewise, sometimes the person we share a home with will feel like "the one thing standing between ourselves and an orderly home."

Because different people have different needs for order and abundance, be sensitive to your spouse and children if they tend to hoard more than you do. If you are cleaner than they are, you might want to consider a recommendation by Victoria Moran. She believes that an ideal way to deal with these kinds of situations is to allow others to keep their own private spaces as messy as they want. For the home's common areas, the person who most values cleanliness may take up the lion's share of the work. Although this might seem unjust, Moran believes that the person who most values cleanliness is the one who will most appreciate it, so it is not unreasonable to expect that they will work a little harder than the others to achieve this goal.

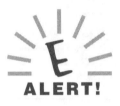

ALERT!

Although the people you live with do have a dramatic effect on the level of organization and cleanliness in your home, don't fall into the temptation of blaming others for the domestic chaos. Instead, work to improve your own habits, and you may be able to inspire those around you to begin to work on theirs.

The Pack Rat Versus the Purger

The old cliché says that opposites attract. This is certainly the case when it comes to home management. In many relationships, a pack rat falls for a purger. The resulting tensions are usually not mentioned in premarital counseling classes. And many couples may feel that they are the only ones who struggle over stuff. But this problem may actually be far more universal than most people realize.

Not only do tensions arise when adults bring different childhood coping mechanisms into a relationship, but sparks can also fly over stuff. While the pack rat feels that it is his duty to hold on to items at any cost, the purger may feel that it is her duty to wage a solo war against clutter.

All is well when the purger is simply sorting through her own items, but should she get carried away (as purgers tend to) and actually begin to impose her habits on the pack rat's territory, you can expect that the pack rat is going to get defensive, if not downright furious.

The pack rat might be willing to purge, but he needs to be given time and space to do it in his own way, without the purger prompting him. Likewise the purger might get tense when the pack rat points out that the purger has just disposed of something that was still needed. The purger might get still more tense if the pack rat begins to exhibit unusual and untrusting behaviors, such as investigating the contents of the dumpster or screening all items on the back porch for signs of immanent removal.

If you are a pack rat who is intimately involved with a purger, or vice versa, keep in mind that your arguments are not really about "stuff." The way that each of you relates to material possessions can point to deep, internal issues that are larger than possessions. As difficult as it can be to see the other person's point of view, keep in mind that you are treading on an emotional land mine when you begin to criticize the way another person relates to the material world. There are genuine differences between people, and it pays to be patient enough to slowly try to understand these distinctions before you act.

Parents and Children

During pregnancy, parents tend to fantasize about the child they will one day hold in their arms. They may imagine that the child will come to them as a blank, impressionable slate, ready to be molded into a miniature version of themselves (retaining all their strong points, of course, while eliminating all negative traits).

For anyone who has had a child, however, this illusion tends to be the very first thing to go, along with one's prepregnancy figure. From the moment they come into the world, children express preferences. Some newborns will sob if you put them in clothes that "don't feel right," such as denim. Some prefer to nurse on only one side; some have very clear ideas about the way they want to be held—facing outward or inward, or slumped over a shoulder. The opinions that are revealed during the newborn phase are just the beginning: your children will continue to manifest preferences through every phase of their lives.

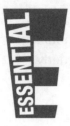

In the book *Parenting with Love and Logic* by Foster Kline and Jim Fay, the authors recommend that parents give their children an opportunity to clean up their toys. If items are routinely left on the floor, parents can remove those items from the house. This action is only to be taken, of course, after warning the child.

And yes, children often have very different ideas than their parents about stuff. The chintziest plastic figure from a McDonald's Happy Meal could be your child's prized possession. The sappy book that grates on your ears with a tinny "electric tune" might just be your child's favorite. The items that you treasure—say a lovely children's book with exquisite illustrations—could mean little to your child. The emotional intensity of the parent-child bond can manifest itself in discussions surrounding the child's belongings. The "what to keep, what to give away" question can provoke surprisingly intense emotions, for both parent and child.

In Chapter 11 you will learn more about how to manage parent-child dynamics when it comes to possessions. This terrain can be almost as gritty as that between partners who are struggling through similar issues.

If you have children, the work of decluttering your home will (like every other area of your life) be a bit more complicated. You'll have to navigate these relationships with respect and gentleness, while still remaining committed to your goal of clutter-free living. As a parent, you have an opportunity to help your child learn how to recognize items of lasting value and to let other items go. You may even be able to teach them how to be generous with their possessions by taking them with you on monthly trips to the Salvation Army.

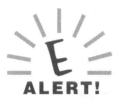

When your children are small, you can freely purge and organize their possessions. As they age, however, it is much better to include them in the process. Help them develop a strategy for their room that works for them, and they will be more likely to cooperate.

If you can cultivate the gift of discernment in your child when she is young, she will not want to live in chaotic and cluttered homes as an adult. Once a person—young or old—learns how good it feels to live in an orderly environment, she rarely chooses to live in clutter.

Solo Organizing

Even if you live by yourself, clutter can still be a problem. While you may not have to navigate the emotional terrain of live-in children and partners, you may also feel a little less motivated to declutter. In the same way that it can be a challenge to cook for one, it can also be a challenge to organize and declutter alone.

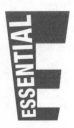

If you are grieving a loss or struggling through a transition, take time to incorporate the change. While you may be forced to make decisions quickly, try your best to pace yourself when possible. Remember that it might be risky to make decisions if you have not yet had a chance to stabilize.

Although you might not have to argue over every item that you wish to purge, it can also be a challenge to make these decisions without another person to serve as a sounding board. Many people live alone not by choice, but as the result of a traumatic experience, such as the death of a spouse. If you are grieving the death of a spouse or a relationship that fell apart, it is normal to experience a lot of emotions surrounding the items that you shared with the other person. Even if you want to organize, you might find that some days you feel utterly incapacitated. Those days, try your best to just take it easy—to weep if necessary—and rest.

After a loss, even if you want to declutter your home, you might find that the mere thought of giving away items is overwhelming. Indeed, if you are grieving or struggling through a transitional period of life, even the simple act of taking the garbage out may seem beyond your capacity. You don't need to make every decision instantly, and you can expect your feelings about your home to change a good deal over the next several months. It may be best not to make any sudden decisions before you're ready.

That said, often the death of a spouse or a change in relationship status will necessitate a move. This move often comes more quickly than a person can anticipate and requires hundreds—sometimes thousands—of decisions about material possessions.

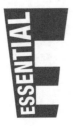

If you are grieving, allow yourself to feel the emotions associated with your possessions. Sometimes, even if you want to purge items, you might need to take things slowly. When you become exhausted, stop for the day. Grieving is some of the hardest work in the world. Cut yourself some slack!

The other side of solo organizing is that, even if you live alone, the work of making a home is still valuable. Even if no one else is there to appreciate your efforts every day, your home environment will nonetheless have a dramatic effect on the way you feel and live in it. The way you feel in your own home can have a ripple effect on the world around you. If you are at peace, others will be more relaxed in your presence. Also, if you can bring more order to your home, you will find it easier to host people there. Chaotic homes are generally less hospitable because they do not create a comfortable space for guests to relax.

Living in the Present

If you live alone, one of the best things you can do is create the home you want to be in, right now. Don't put off living simply because the situation you're in is not what you imagined it could be. Instead, devote yourself to making your home a refuge that you long to return to at the end of the day.

In the book *Shelter for the Spirit*, Victoria Moran writes about her experience creating a home after her husband died. She was still a young woman with a young daughter to care for, and it was challenging to find ways to embrace her current situation. She writes about the temptation to delay life—and to put off experiencing the enjoyment our homes could give us—until we've found ourselves in our dream situation or home.

Perhaps you want to be married and have children someday, but you haven't found yourself in the right situation. The best thing you can do is to start living well now, in the circumstances you've been given, with the resources you have. Only when you begin to live in the now will you be able to prepare for and enjoy the possibilities as they present themselves to you in each moment.

Chapter 2

Feng Shui and the Spiritual Dimensions of Space

For thousands of years, people around the world have cultivated an awareness of the spiritual dimensions of space. Many religions have a concept of "sanctifying space" through house blessings, prayers, and energy balancing. In contemporary society, people are increasingly seeking ways to heal, bless, and transform not just their physical environments, but their spiritual environments as well. This chapter will explore ways to sanctify space—everything from feng shui to traditional Christian house blessings.

What Is Feng Shui?

Feng shui, pronounced "fung shway," is the study of energy and how it affects people positively or negatively. Feng shui is an ancient Chinese practice that was developed by agrarian people who recognized their dependence on the natural forces of the world. Feng shui, by integrating the Taoist search for balance and the Buddhist quest for harmony, seeks to incorporate these principles into the home.

Energy Flow

One of the primary principles of feng shui is that you want the energy in your home to connect with the natural life-forces outdoors. You must allow the energy to flow freely through your home, and not hamper it by having excess clutter or by leaving things broken, including damaged or cracked windows. According to this belief system, energy flows best along curving spaces—ovals and circles are preferable to jutting corners and straight lines.

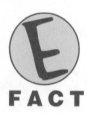

FACT

In English, *feng shui* means "the way of wind and water" or "the natural forces of the universe." The ancient Chinese lived by these forces. Europeans call these forces "geomancy," and Hawaiians and Native Americans practice their own methods of energy balancing. The fundamental concepts behind feng shui have been studied and explored throughout history by people around the world.

According to the principles of feng shui, you can transform your living and work environments by making them more attuned to the life forces around you. Feng shui is disrupted by chaos. An orderly home is more conducive to positive energy flow than a chaotic one.

Many people are initially quite skeptical about feng shui. Although some of the principles might not resonate with you, many of the ideas will likely mesh with your own intuition, as if they explain something that has never before been clearly articulated.

Victoria Moran was also initially unsure of what to make of feng shui. She writes, "When I first heard about feng shui, it sounded like a Far Eastern rendition of avoiding black cats . . . Nevertheless, many of the principles are clearly in keeping with contemporary psychology. Cheerful people are healthier and more productive than glum ones, and a pleasing atmosphere in the home or office does contribute to happiness."

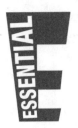

While some of the ideas associated with feng shui may seem a little odd and unrealistic for your own space, others follow the lines of common sense. Many of the ideas associated with feng shui seemed to be fundamental and universal concepts that can make sense to people in any life circumstance and of any religious persuasion.

While feng shui used to be thought of as a wacky invention of the New Age movement, people are increasingly becoming aware of the spiritual dimensions of space and the value of living intentionally in one's own home. Certain arrangements of furniture and home orientations evoke emotions— clutter can cause a feeling of helplessness, broken things can make you feel depressed, and dark, dingy spaces can oppress your spirit. The feng shui principle that curving lines are more conducive to a healthy and aesthetically pleasing space, for example, make sense to anyone who has lived in a shoebox apartment.

First Principles

According to the principles of feng shui, the first steps in healing the space in which you dwell are quite concrete: get rid of the clutter, fix the broken things, and bring a little more light to your space through the use of mirrors. Clutter is trapped energy that has far-reaching effects, physically, mentally, and spiritually. It is believed that all forms of household clutter can keep you trapped in the past, congest your body, and make you feel lethargic and fatigued.

According to the principles of feng shui, when you clear out clutter you release negative emotions, generate positive energy, and carve-out space to do the things you most hope to do in your home or work environment. The idea that clutter holds people back from realizing their potential seems to be a universal belief, held not just by practitioners of feng shui, but by professional organizers as well.

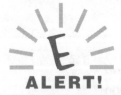

ALERT!

One of feng shui's primary concerns about clutter is that it is not forward looking. Clutter is often a way of clinging to the past and can be crippling to a person who wants to take steps to move toward the future. According to this philosophy, by getting rid of clutter, you create space for new possibilities.

Healing the Home

After you've begun the work of decluttering your environment, take a mental inventory of broken things in your home and garden and begin to make a focused effort to fix these things. It is also wise to clean dirty spaces. You might be especially mindful of windows, because according to these principles, windows are the eyes of the chi (the life-force energy) and they affect your mental clarity. This is one of those intuitive feng shui ideas. Anyone who spent a winter staring out of a streaked and dirty window knows how irritating the smudges become over time. Dirty windows strain your eyes and you have to focus to see out. They also can feel like a reproach every time the sunlight exposes all that dirt.

On a more basic level, smudged or cracked windows can interfere with your experience of light and beauty—instead of seeing your lovely garden, you might just see those flecks of dirt. The dirt might make you feel burdened and worried with thoughts like, "How am I going to tackle *that?*" These small things can detract from your experience of home, and can have a significant negative impact on your mood.

Feng shui teaches that the systems of your home correspond to your bodily systems. You might have been able to guess that plumbing corresponds to your body's digestive system, so those who believe in this model would say that it is wise to repair leaky faucets and clogged drains promptly if you wish to keep your digestive system in good working order. Likewise, the electrical system in your home corresponds to your neurological system.

Feng shui also offers many principles related to organizing and decorating. One is that the main door represents the home's mouth of the chi. Symbolically, this is how the entire chi enters your home, so you want to keep this entrance clear, open, and clutter-free. The front door should also be large and easily accessible. Your home is best placed level to or just above the sidewalk, and the front hedges should be kept neatly trimmed. Practitioners of feng shui also teach that a fountain in front of the home is an excellent way to increase "flowing money energy" and draw it into your home. Ever notice all the mansions with fountains out front? The water element is a universal symbol for wealth and prosperity.

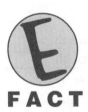

Feng shui practitioners believe that it is not ideal to enter a bathroom and immediately see the toilet. This idea seems to mesh with common sense—a toilet set into an alcove is far more pleasing on the eye and peaceful to use than one placed in the center of the room.

When Feng Shui Falls Short

There are some ideas associated with feng shui that might run counter to your own intuitive sense about how you wish to organize your home. For example, it is considered good feng shui to have your desk facing a door. But for many people, a view out the window is preferable to a glimpse of the door. In these kinds of situations, follow your own intuition, even when they run counter to a philosophy such as feng shui that offers valuable insights.

Ten Basic Principles

There are ten basic principles of feng shui that are useful for those who wish to incorporate some of these ideas into their lives. Many of the ideas of feng shui may resonate with you, even if you subscribe to other belief systems.

These principles are:

1. **Clear the clutter.** Besides taking up physical space, clutter can block new opportunities and keep you locked in the past. By clearing out your home, you create space for a future full of possibilities.

2. **Keep the front entrance of your home well maintained.** The entrance area of your home is where it all begins. Try to keep it clear, clutter-free, and well-lit. Just as HGTV and other television channels promote shows such as *Curb Appeal* that are intended to increase the value of your home by transforming first impressions, the practitioners of feng shui have long believed that the front door is central to the home.

3. **Allow energy to flow freely.** Energy should be able to flow through your home to promote good health and harmony. Avoid interfering with this flow with clutter or awkwardly placed furniture.

4. **Contain the energy.** Energy needs to be able to flow around the house in order to nourish you. Avoid situations that allow energy to rush through the house and quickly escape. The back door should not be directly aligned with the front door, for example. If this is the case in your home, consider hanging wind chimes to moderate and redirect the flow of energy.

5. **Make sure everything works.** Stay on top of maintenance issues. Fix items quickly and keep your surroundings as clean as possible. It is believed that every job left half-done somehow reflects an aspect of your life that is incomplete and needs attention.

6. **Be aware of energy issues.** According to feng shui, distortions in the electromagnic fields can impact your mental clarity over a period of time. Feng shui experts believe that sometimes energy needs to be "rebalanced" by a trained professional.

7. **Be aware of the images and symbols in your home.** Your choice of art, for example, is considered a message from your subconscious. Look around your home to determine what kinds of messages you may have unwittingly projected into your space. Consider changing your art to more consciously reflect your desires for the future.

8. **Create a quiet sanctuary in your bedroom.** Your bedroom should be an oasis of peace and serenity. Attention to your sleeping environment may help you to sleep more deeply at night. Clear the clutter out of this

space, and avoid using your bedroom for any stressful activity, such as working, arguing, or balancing your checkbook.

9. **Make the kitchen a center of calmness.** The kitchen is often considered the hub of family life. Make this room a contained area where you can prepare meals in peace. According to the principles of feng shui, the atmosphere of your kitchen will permeate the food that you prepare and serve.

10. **Love your home and it will love you.** Think of your home as a living being. If you care for it and nourish it, it will in turn support and nurture you.

If you integrate some of the principles of feng shui into your home, you may find that you can rest better, live better, and entertain more freely in your space.

Hiring a Consultant

Although it is fairly simple to grasp the basic principles of feng shui, it can take years to truly understand its underlying principles. Some people who intuitively resonate with the principles of feng shui and want to learn more can hire a professional feng shui consultant who can come into their home and offer practical tips for increasing energy flow and releasing trapped negative emotions.

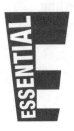

The concept of "sanctifying space" is present in many cultures around the world. The basic concept is that we can have a dramatic effect on our environment when we learn to see it with spiritual eyes. This idea is based on the belief that space is not necessarily neutral as people most often assume, but the very air can be charged with positive or negative spiritual elements.

Unless you are building a new home from scratch, the basic structures of your home can't be easily modified. Obviously, it will not be possible to change the orientation of your home or move the entrance. That said, feng shui offers practical, doable ideas for using smaller objects to change your space. These "cures" involve the use of symbolic items, color, and repositioning of furniture. A consultant can help diagnose the quirks in your home and help identify solutions.

The best way to find a local feng shui expert is through a referral from someone you know and trust. You can visit the International Feng Shui Guild at *www.internationalfengshuiguild.org*. This group hopes to promote the use, practice, and teachings of feng shui.

A professional feng shui practitioner might offer you advice in these areas:

- Furniture placement
- Methods to cultivate or enhance certain areas of your life
- The best rooms in your home or office for specific activities
- Ideas for optimizing the use of colors
- Increasing the beauty of outdoor environmental designs
- Creating a sanctuary or meditation space within your home
- Correct positioning of home-office implements
- Ideas to improve the flow of chi through the front entrance of your home
- Ideal places for feng shui cures, such as chimes, mirrors, lights, fountains, candles, and mobiles

The cost of hiring a professional feng shui consultant varies according to location and other factors, so be sure to determine fees and services covered before bringing the consultant into your home.

Room to Pray or Meditate

George Bernandos (as quoted in *Wabi Sabi: The Art of Everyday Life* by Diane Durston) wrote, "You owe it to everyone you love (including yourself) to find pockets of tranquility in your busy world." Many world religions acknowledge the need to create these quiet pockets in the midst of the busyness of home.

Within Eastern Orthodox Christianity, it is a common practice to create an "icon corner." An icon corner contains icons—two-dimensional stylized images of the saints and Christ. Families will often select icons that are specifically connected to family members who reside in the home.

Traditionally, Orthodox children are given a saint's name seven days after they are born. A family's icon corner is likely to contain an icon of Jesus, one of Mary, and icons associated with each family member's saint. In this way, an icon corner both follows a certain convention and leaves room for personalization. Icon corners can be located in any room, but many families place them in their dining rooms, as that is an area where everyone gathers daily. Small icon corners can also be useful in children's rooms. They can help a child feel protected even when she is alone and wakeful in her room at night.

Believers most often place their icon corners on an Eastern wall, because this is the traditional orientation of churches, symbolically linked to the idea that the sun rises from the East and the Rising of the Son (or Christ) is central to Christian belief. The Eastern Orthodox also often keep a small lamp burning in their icon corner, called a lampada. This small lamp most often consists of a wick attached to a cork circle and floating in olive oil, which burns safely and cleanly. Some people keep their lampada burning at all times as a reminder that God is present everywhere and fills all things, and so that believers are called to remain alert and available to God.

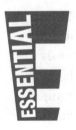

You might place a rug or comfortable chair before the icons or altar. If a prayer or meditation area is inviting, a person is more inclined to linger there. Some people also add plants, fresh flowers, or photographs. These objects can serve as a link to loved ones, and help to bring elements from the natural world into the prayer space.

A Spiritual Hearth

A prayer corner can also serve as a "spiritual hearth" of sorts. This area does not have to be experienced in solitude. Here, a family can come together for prayers or thanksgiving or simply just to be quiet. By intentionally creating a space for prayer and meditation, you are far more likely to find ways to integrate spirituality into your home.

A Space of Healing

You might find that your prayer or meditation corner can also become a place of mental, and possibly even physical, healing. Our brains and bodies are often wearied and ragged by the end of the day. As Victoria Moran writes in *Shelter for the Spirit*, "Meditation and prayer provide a restorative atmosphere for physical and mental healing. They are not a cure per se, but they allow healing to happen, the way a home filled with books does not teach a child to read but provides the raw material for him to become a reader."

It can be easy to forget the spiritual dimensions of space unless you are intentional about creating "holy places" that call you back to a deep, fertile quiet. In these corners of home, you create the possibility of wholeness, wellness, and hope. These gifts extend beyond your own soul and body to every life you come in contact with. As the Russian saint Seraphim of Serov said, "Acquire inner peace and thousands around you will be saved."

A Hospitable Home

Another way to attend to the spiritual dimensions of home is to seek to be intentionally hospitable, to open your home to welcome, feed, and nurture both friends and strangers. One philosophy of homemaking that is slowly catching on in American society is wabi-sabi. This ancient Japanese philosophy is related to creating spaces that are uncluttered, adorned with weathered or handmade items, and intentionally hospitable. The elaborate rituals related to the Japanese tea ceremony are expressive of the wabi-sabi mentality, which has at its heart consideration for others.

In *The Wabi-Sabi House: The Japanese Art of Imperfect Beauty*, Robyn Griggs Lawrence says that the key to hospitality is being attentive to the needs of others: "If it's cold, greet guests with a hot drink and invite them into a room warmed by a roaring fire. If it's warm, play tropical music and pass out fans. Keep their drinks filled. Watch for wallflowers and spend as much time as you can with them . . . Bear in mind Sen no Rikyu's Seventh rule of tea: Always be mindful of guests."

If your home is orderly and the atmosphere peaceful, it will be a place where people want to linger. After guests leave and dishes are being stacked in the dishwasher, the blessing of their presence seems to linger in the home. Some people believe that hospitable homes don't just strengthen those who visit the home, but also nourish those who dwell there daily. As Kurt Vonnegut said, "The most daring thing is to create stable communities where the terrible disease of loneliness can be cured."

The theme of hospitality is present throughout the New Testament. In the book of Hebrews it says, "Be mindful to entertain strangers because in so doing some have entertained angels unaware." This passage probably refers back to the Old Testament story of the hospitality of Abraham, through which Abraham and Sarah were likely more blessed than their guests.

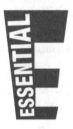

One way to enjoy your guests more is to allow them to help. Especially if you'll be having a large group over, invite a few friends to help with the cooking and preparations beforehand. When people offer to help, take them up on it so that you can spend more time with your guests.

The theme of hospitality is also present in the ancient Eastern Orthodox wedding service. During the course of this service, a prayer is said over the couple "that they will be blessed with wheat, wine, and oil so that they can give to others in need." The notion of hospitality is based on the idea that gifts are intended to be shared. By generously sharing your space with others, you not only help others, you can help yourself and help your home to achieve its full potential.

As Victoria Moran writes in *Shelter for the Spirit*: "Gather some people around you and let your experiences blend with theirs. They may bring flowers or a candle or a bottle of wine, but those gifts aren't the ones that will live in your home as long as you do. The gift of each individual's presence is that lasting, though. Adding the good cheer of friends to objects that inspire you, simplified space, delicious food and lovingly maintained surroundings will result in the sort of space your soul will want to come home to."

House Blessings

Another way to increase the goodness in your home is to do a house blessing. Many cultures around the world have concepts of house blessings. Within Christianity, house blessings occur most often in the Eastern Orthodox, Roman Catholic, and Anglican churches.

Spiritual Transformation

The basic idea of a house blessing is that space can be transformed through prayer. In most cases, blessed water from the church will be sprinkled through the home by a priest while members of the family and close friends follow the priest and sing. A house blessing can create an opportunity to remember every gift that has been given to those who dwell in the home, and also to remember that the family is much larger than the small group of people who dwell there.

Families stretch back generations and incorporate both the living and the dead. This is why prayers are traditionally said for those on both sides of the grave. Families can also extend beyond the confines of biology to embrace friends and the wider community. A house blessing can help anchor people in this larger reality.

Preparing for a House Blessing

Before a house blessing, families clean their homes to a shine and prepare a meal, snacks, or dessert for those who will come. The act of preparing the home can be a joyful time, full of anticipation, hope, and gratitude. During the house blessing, prayers may also be said over each area of the home, as a way of consecrating specific rooms to specific purposes. In more elaborate house blessings, crosses will also be drawn with olive oil on the four main walls of the home. Within the Eastern Orthodox Church, an elaborate house blessing service is often performed when a family moves into a home, and then smaller house blessings will be performed each January—

after the feast of Theophany, when water is blessed and Christ's baptism is remembered.

The smaller annual services are a way of continually attending to the spiritual atmosphere of the home, praying for those who dwell there, and infusing the physical space with a sense of spiritual purpose. This might be considered a form of "spiritual housekeeping." House blessings are also a way for communities to celebrate all the gifts that have been given and the way that all these gifts come together in the home.

Chapter 3

The Cost of Clutter

Clutter drains your pocketbook as well as your spirit. Those who live in over-stuffed homes are more likely to lose important paperwork, such as credit card bills and checks. When there is too much clutter and important items disappear, you might be forced to run to the store for something you already own. This chapter explores the hidden cost of clutter and some ways to sell your way out of it.

Time Is Money

While you may think that the clutter in your home costs nothing to keep, most people do lose money on clutter. Not only might having too many possessions keep you from being able to find the things that you need when you need them, but sometimes when items can't be found quickly, you might be tempted to rush to the store to replace the item.

Not only does clutter affect your home life, it can also spill into your professional life. Those who lose things because of unmanaged clutter may suffer a loss in credibility as well. If you are a professional who is regularly late to meetings or misses deadlines because of misplaced proposals, notes, and the like, you can expect that your business will suffer because people will be wary of trusting you with important documents and projects.

Not only does clutter (and the resulting chaos) undermine your reputation, it can cause you to waste precious energy and time searching for things that could be kept in an easily accessible spot. This kind of chaos can also prevent you from being fully present to the work at hand. Instead of being able to focus on your current task, your mind rushes in a thousand different directions.

When you are distracted by piles of clutter and the nagging feeling that you'll never be able to get them under control, work takes longer and is generally less impressive in the end. Focus comes with an ability to see what is essential and central.

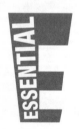

Another problem with clutter and disorganization is that it may interfere with your ability to pay bills on time. Late fees and increased APRs on credit cards can greatly increase your cost of living over the years. Not only that, but missed bills can negatively affect your credit rating. Nobody needs these kinds of marks against him—especially if the problem is not actually lack of funds, but rather lack of organization.

The other area that will cost you in terms of clutter is your home—if at any point you want to sell your home, the first thing you'll need to do is purge the clutter. Clutter can greatly detract from the ambiance and appearance of your home. Realtors generally believe that an uncluttered home will create a far more favorable impression for potential buyers—buyers need to be able to see into the farthest reaches of your closets. They also must quickly see the innate beauty of your home, which can easily be obscured by clutter. Likewise, the respect and love you devote to your home by keeping it tidy and uncluttered communicates to potential buyers that your home is worth their energy, love, and money.

Sitting on a Gold Mine?

The bad news is that clutter is costly. The good news, however, is that hidden in your clutter there may be many items of value. When you dig deep into chaotic drawers and closets you might be surprised at the things you find—attractive clothes, important records, long-lost love letters. You never know what will turn up; the clutter could conceal items of both financial and emotional value.

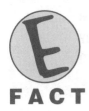

FACT

In recent years, people have shown renewed interest in digging up old items and seeing what they're worth. From that painting that used to hang above Grandma's couch to the vase you got at a garage sale, you might find some truly valuable items tucked away in the dark corners of your home. Anything that doesn't have sentimental value that can be sold might be worth some money.

As you sort through the clutter, you'll probably find items that have been missing for some time. Perhaps you'll find that you have plenty of clothes that you like and that fit, and you won't need to replace your winter wardrobe after all. Perhaps you'll find your older child's snowsuit and boots and you can pass them on to your younger child instead of being forced to purchase something new. A few lucky souls may even find gift certificates they'd forgotten about, or valuable items such as a working scanner or fax machine that can be sold online for a decent price. While your clutter may be costly for you to keep, it may have value that you haven't yet discovered. Especially now that items are widely sold online, you can often recoup at least some of your initial investment.

Have a Yard Sale

One way to earn a bit of extra cash through getting rid of your unwanted stuff is to hold a yard sale or garage sale. Before embarking on this type of project, know what you're getting into and plan accordingly. A yard sale is an excellent opportunity to sell unwanted furniture, knickknacks, clothing, used sports equipment, jewelry, collectibles, and other personal and/or household items. Keep in mind, however, that at best, you'll probably receive only a fraction of what you originally paid for the items you're selling. People who attend yard sales do so in search of bargains. If they find something they want, they will likely negotiate for the lowest possible price.

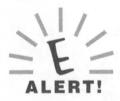

ALERT!

Yard sales can involve a significant investment of time. If you are in a rush to get your home in order, you may not want to divert your energy in this way, especially because most items can only be sold for a fraction of their original cost.

After sorting through all of the rooms in your home, determine whether you have enough stuff to sell to make organizing, promoting, and actually holding a yard sale worthwhile. You may want to ask a few of your neighbors and friends to participate and sell some of their unwanted belongings as well.

Taking Inventory

Take inventory of the items you plan to sell. Make a point to clean up items so that they're in the best possible condition. Then set prices for the items you plan to sell, knowing that the price you set will be a starting point for a negotiation.

If you're selling clothing, give the items fair prices, keeping age and wear in mind as you determine their value. If you're selling collectibles, consider a price that's about half of what the book value is. For other types of items, set prices you think are fair, based on value and condition. You can always lower your prices during the actual sale.

One way to ensure that your prices are market appropriate is to attend several other yard sales in your community and see what prices other people are asking for similar things. Make sure you stick price tags on all of your items. You may also want to post signs stating that you're willing to negotiate. It's also an excellent strategy to offer a "buy two, get one free" offer on items such as books, videos, CDs, video games, and some types of collectibles (e.g., trading cards).

Promoting Your Event

Advertising is critical for drawing a crowd. Send a notice to local newspapers stating the date, time, location, and types of items to be sold. Most community newspapers have a local calendar or events section in which yard sales are listed, sometimes free of charge. You can also take advantage of paid classified advertising, or in many cities you can advertise for free via craigslist (*www.craigslist.org*).

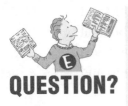

QUESTION?

How do I price my items for a yard sale?
People often overvalue their own possessions. A realistic price for a used item that is still in good condition would be between 10 percent and 30 percent of the original cost. If your sale lasts two days, drop prices even further on the second day so that you can move more items.

As for other forms of advertising, nothing is more important than plastering your community with signs. Several days before the event, post signs in your community—on lampposts, in store windows (with permission), on community bulletin boards, and in supermarkets. If you'll be selling special items, such as a rare coin collection or children's clothes, highlight this information on your signs. You also want to clearly display the date, time, and location of your event. If possible, create signs that are waterproof. Most hardware stores sell plastic "Yard Sale" or "Garage Sale" signs; you can use a permanent marker to write in the important details. It's also helpful to announce the reason for the sale. For example, your sign may say "Moving Sale."

Post your signs in high-traffic areas within a two-mile radius of your home. Your signs should answer these basic questions (but not necessarily in this order): who, what, where, when, and why. Remember to make the largest signs possible and make them easy to read. Make sure someone looking at your signs will learn the important facts quickly.

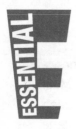

Also don't overlook the power of the Internet to promote your event. Local chat rooms and message forums are an ideal place to share information about your upcoming yard sale. You can also use the Internet to seek out information about putting together a sale.

On the day of the sale, hang balloons in front of your home and at the end of your street (if possible) to draw the attention of customers. As you begin to display your items, think about setting up a large bin or table and offering a few items for free. Select items that you want to get rid of, but that you don't think people will pay money for. Not only is offering a few items for free a nice gesture, it also helps create a buyer-friendly atmosphere and will help reduce shoplifting.

Whenever possible, display your items on tables, bookshelves, or portable clothing racks. Try to keep the items organized and readily accessible. Don't make people dig through piles of stuff to find what they're looking for. Also, divide up your items into categories. For example, set aside separate areas for used sports equipment, kitchen items, clothing, CDs and videos, furniture, collectibles, and books.

Selling Items Online

If you have a few expensive items to sell, such as furniture or collectibles, consider selling those items online, using an online auction service such as eBay (*www.ebay.com*), Half.com (*www.half.ebay.com*, or craigslist (*www.craigslist.org*).

An online auction is just like a live auction: people bid on an object, which is sold to the highest bidder. A potential buyer participates by bidding on an item that a seller has listed. The person who has offered the highest bid at close of auction wins the right to purchase the item at that price.

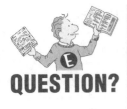

QUESTION?

Can I get someone to sell my items online for me?
Sure! If selling your items online feels like too much of a headache, consider using a service, such as "Sell it on eBay," that will price, list, and ship your items for you. These middlemen always take a commission, but you may not actually lose money because their experience helps them to get the best price.

Make sure you list your items under the appropriate category within the online auction site. eBay, for example, offers a variety of main categories and subcategories, such as antiques and art, clothing and accessories, dolls and bears, jewelry, and so on.

When preparing a listing, have the following information available. Also keep in mind that many potential buyers will be less likely to want to purchase an item from you if you have not posted a digital photo of the item.

- **Title:** Include a brief, thoughtful title that accurately describes the item you are selling. A title that's easy to understand will make your item easier for bidders to find.
- **Description:** Describe the product in detail. The more detail you provide, the more confidence you'll inspire among the bidders.
- **Sales policies:** Select the types of payment you're willing to accept. These could include cashier's checks, money orders, cash, personal

checks, credit cards, or an online payment option such as PayPal. (PayPal is an ideal option because the cash will be available almost immediately, although you will have to create a PayPal account.)

- **Shipping options:** Decide whether you or the buyer pays the shipping costs. Decide when the item will ship, either upon receipt of payment or immediately after the auction closes. You might also want to save yourself the hassle of shipping and say "pick-up only." Local Web sites, such as craigslist.org, are ideal for the pick-up-only option.
- **Quantity of item:** If you have more than one of the same item, and you would like to sell each one individually (in which case there may be several buyers), consider listing each product separately.
- **Starting price:** Enter the price that will be used to start the auction.
- **Length of auction:** Determine how many days the auction will last.

It's also very important to be completely honest about any flaws or damage on any items you're trying to sell. If you attempt to gloss over any problems with the item, you may get a very unhappy buyer. This buyer might then post negative feedback next to your name on eBay, and you could lose credibility. A loss of credibility will negatively affect your future sales.

Selling to Antique Stores or Consignment Shops

If you only have a few items you're interested in selling, and these items (such as antiques, jewelry, furniture, or collectibles) have significant value, consider working directly with an antique store or consignment shop to sell them. These shops may pay you a negotiated price up-front, or you may have to wait until the consignment shop sells your items before you receive your money. Either way, you can potentially earn cash for your unwanted items. Check the Yellow Pages for a list of consignment shops and/or antique dealers in your area. Assuming you know that the items you're hoping to sell are valuable, get them appraised independently so you know exactly what they're worth before negotiating a sale price.

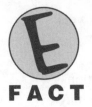

FACT

You'll find a variety of consignment shop agreements. Some charge a straight commission (as much as 50 percent of the purchase price on items sold). Other shops charge space rental plus a commission, while still others charge a flat space-rental fee. For items that don't sell quickly, some shops require that you remove the merchandise or mark it down within a specified time. Be sure to ask what the policy is for the consignment shop you are considering. Also, make sure to get the terms in writing.

Donating Items to Charity

No matter what items you have to get rid of, one possibility is to donate them to a local charity. Depending on the charity, you can donate used clothing, furniture, appliances, vehicles, canned (or prepackaged) food items, old sports equipment, eyeglasses, and just about anything else that others might be able to use.

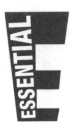

ESSENTIAL

Take care that any item you donate to charity is in acceptable condition. Clothing that is stained, torn, or otherwise damaged should not be donated. Out of respect to these organizations and to the people who patronize them, only donate items that you would not be ashamed to own.

While you won't receive cash for making a donation to a charity, you can take a tax deduction if the charity you donate your stuff to is legitimate and provides you with a receipt.

Here is a listing of some charities that might be interested in your castaways:

- The Women's Alliance (*www.thewomensalliance.org*) is a national not-for-profit membership alliance of independent community-based groups that increase the employability of low-income women. Assistance provided to these women includes donated professional attire, career-skills training, and a range of support services from dental care to health and wellness programs.
- Dress for Success (*www.dressforsuccess.org*) is a not-for-profit organization that helps low-income women transition into the work force. Each client receives one suit for her interview and a second suit when she lands a job.
- The Salvation Army (*www.salvationarmy.org*) is an international movement, collecting a wide variety of items and selling them cheaply. They also provide jobs and training those who work in their centers.
- Volunteers of America (*www.voa.org*) is a national, not-for-profit, faith-based organization providing local service programs and the opportunity for individual and community involvement in about 300 communities across the country.
- Goodwill Industries (*www.goodwill.org*) is one of the world's largest not-for-profit providers of employment and training services for people with disabilities and other conditions, such as welfare dependency, illiteracy, criminal history, and homelessness.

Should you have old computers or computer equipment on hand, consider donating them to a worthy charity. In Julie Morgenstern's book *Organizing from the Inside Out*, she lists several charities that will refurbish old computers and ship them overseas to needy children.

Here is a listing of a few of these charities:

- The National Cristina Foundation (*www.cristina.org*)
- World Computer Exchange (*www.worldcomputerexchange.org*)
- Computers for Schools (*www.pcsforschools.org*)

Keep in mind that computers are unsafe for landfills and should be disposed of properly. Don't try to sneak "techno-trash" in with your regular garbage. Check with your city's recycling department to see what kind of recycling options are available. Many cities offer a "blue bag" or pick-up service for electrical items. This will ensure that your items are recycled or disposed of properly. Even if you can't recoup your initial investment, nothing is completely wasted when you make an ecologically conscious decision.

Chapter 4

Starting Small

The Chinese philosopher Lao Tzu wrote, "A journey of a thousand miles begins with a single step." This is true for interior journeys as well as the larger external ones. This chapter offers a sampling of "baby steps" to help you on the journey. This is not about achieving perfection; rather, it is about learning to walk, to take small, concrete steps toward realistic goals that can make your home more serene, inviting, and orderly.

4

Check Your Expectations

One of the biggest temptations in almost every area of life is the impulse to try to take on too much, too fast. This is a huge problem when it comes to homes. Instead of trying to tackle organizational problems in small, manageable steps, people are often tempted to try to take on the whole project at once—to plan a kitchen remodel while organizing the bathroom, sweeping the garage, and vacuuming the living room.

When too much is taken on too fast, people quickly experience "crash-and burn" syndrome. One can quickly become discouraged, paralyzed, and exhausted, collapsing on the sofa and looking around with despair. But it doesn't have to be this way!

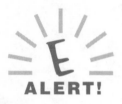
ALERT!

According to Julie Morgenstern, many people put off organizing simply because they imagine that the task will be too time consuming. Try to generate a realistic estimation of the time that each project might take you, and schedule your projects accordingly.

By keeping your expectations in check—and generating only small, manageable goals, such as to spend five minutes a day sorting the bedroom closet—you are more likely to keep going, even when you feel tired. After all, small, achievable goals don't weigh on you as heavily as larger ones can. You know that your goal is realistic when it feels doable. A sense of despair is a good sign that your goals are too lofty and that they need to be cut back down to size.

Overcoming Resistance

Stephen Pressfield's book *The War of Art* defines "Resistance" as the universal derailing force that seeks to undo us the moment we attempt to move to a higher plane in art, academics, relationships, and life. If Resistance had a voice, it would say things like, "You can't, you can't, you can't. You're not smart enough, organized enough, savvy enough."

If you are attempting to bring order to your home, you can expect to experience some Resistance. It can come from the inside or from the outside. You might doubt yourself, and others might question your motives, especially if they are losing the war against Resistance in their own lives. Remember—it is far easier for other people to point out the flaws in your plan than it is for them to wage their own battles.

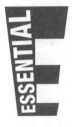

Marla Cilley (the FlyLady) has these words to say about becoming realistic: "Perfectionism will keep you from ever getting out of the CHAOS (Can't Have Anyone Over Syndrome). This process of baby steps is all about progress, not perfection."

According to Pressfield, when you feel overly critical of other people, that is a good sign that you need to stop focusing on others and channel your energies into waging your own battles. Perhaps home organizing seems too menial for these battles to be fierce. But the battles you wage on the home front are every bit as real and significant as the ones that are waged out there in the "real world." In fact, because a home is so closely linked to a sense of well-being and peace of mind, the steps you take at home can, to some extent, predetermine your success (or lack of it) in the outside world.

The Problem with Perfectionism

Perfectionism can paralyze. As soon as you realize all there is to do and all that you hope to accomplish, you can quickly become overwhelmed. Instead of trying to do everything, Pressfield recommends that you just seek to combat Resistance for a little bit every day. He recommends taking small, concrete steps that are not focused on outcomes. Instead of seeking to tackle all of your projects, he advises, just fight Resistance a little bit each day. Even if you can't make your home perfect, you can certainly make it better.

One Life or Two?

"Most of us have two lives," writes Pressfield. "The life you live, and the unlived life within us. Between the two stands Resistance." It could also be said that most people have two homes—the home you dream of living in and the home you actually inhabit. Although economics and other factors may keep you from purchasing your "dream home," it might be possible, in small, concrete ways, to bridge some of the gaps between dreams and reality just by organizing and ordering the home you actually do have, right now. If you can bring order and serenity to your home, your contentment will increase. You might even discover that you don't actually *need* all the things you imagine you do. Just do the best you can with what you have in the present moment, recognizing that your resources (time, money, energy) are finite, but if you keep taking baby steps, your possibilities will expand.

The Five-Minute Pickup

The FlyLady offers this simple directive. Instead of trying to tackle all household chores in one fell swoop, try a five-minute pickup. This means that you set a timer for five minutes, or another short, realistic time span, and then rush around the house picking up things as quickly as you possibly can. This technique is fun and fast and will help alleviate some of the drudgery of cleaning and organizing.

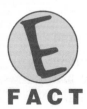

FACT

A variation on the five-minute pickup game is to play it with your children and let them each have a bag or basket. You set the timer and they race around the house collecting as many items that need to be put away as they can. When the timer goes off, whoever has the most items "wins." Then the timer is set again and everyone scrambles to get everything in their baskets put away before the next ding.

It can become a race against the clock as you seek to restore order in a minimal amount of time. It can also help curb the perfectionism that so often haunts household projects, because you just can't afford to demand perfection from yourself when you're trying to beat the clock. The other great benefit of a quick pickup is that it can show you how simple it can be to tidy up. Finally, this method frees us from one of the great temptations that can sabotage our efforts—nostalgia.

Keep Moving

Often, when you begin to tackle a pile of paper you come across things that you want to study and read—old letters, old photos, and ancient report cards. While these items can be fun to peruse, you need to remember that during the five-minute pickup, nostalgia is your enemy. It will slow you down and prevent you from being objective about clutter.

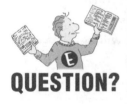

QUESTION?

How can I keep myself from sifting through all those nostalgic items I find?
If decluttering puts you in a nostalgic mood and you want to pick up the pace instead of reading all those old letters and cards, create a box for items to go through before bed or over coffee in the morning. Promise yourself that you'll eventually give these items the time they deserve, but for now you'll simply focus on organizing.

As you go through your possessions, make sure that you remain focused on your goals. Professional housekeepers are able to make a living because they are not emotionally invested in the items they clean. They don't stop to write back to a long-lost friend in the middle of the workday or to peruse old photo albums. Because they know that the clock is ticking, they don't waste time. If you only allow yourself to work for a predetermined amount of time, you might be better able to focus on the work at hand and to accomplish your goals.

Be Positive

Another way to increase the fun of this activity is to introduce some kind of reward. You might consider putting a pot of coffee on to brew. As the aromatic coffee sputters in the pot, you rush around trying to create order. You promise yourself that as soon as the coffee is ready, you can sit and relax with a steaming cup of coffee in your orderly home.

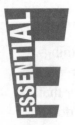

Julie Morgenstern recommends using before and after photos as a way to celebrate a job well done. These photos will help you to remember how far you've come and what is possible if you just devote some time and energy to each room in your home.

Eventually, you might find that order has it own rewards, but when you're trying to develop positive habits, it can be helpful to attach rewards to the tasks you dread, so that instead of thinking "No pain, no gain," you will be more inclined to think of your tasks in a positive way.

Avoiding the Credit Card Mentality

One of the greatest enemies to clutter-free living is a set of credit cards. Those little pieces of plastic might be standing between you and an orderly, uncluttered home. Many of the expensive (and not-so-expensive) items that you bring into your home actually add to the clutter and chaos instead of increasing the beauty.

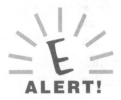

Credit cards are dangerous in a few ways. The first way, which is a bit more cosmic than concrete, is that credit cards create illusions. They create the illusion that a person needs to own bigger and better things than their budget permits. This attitude usually leads to debt and complicates life.

According to Victoria Moran in *Shelter for the Spirit*, if you insist on quality and you only pay cash for your purchases, it will take more time to accumulate things. If you live more intentionally in your space, it may be easier for you to limit clutter and make good decisions about what to keep and what to get rid of. Likewise, if you pay cash and make your purchases slowly, you are more likely to enjoy them for a longer time. Impulse purchases often cause regret later on.

The more you dwell in the concrete realm, the better prepared you are to grapple with the concrete, physical realities of life. Often, you don't need a new fridge to keep your perishables in order—you merely need to keep the fridge you do have in order. You often do not need custom "closet organizers" to set your clothing aright. Instead, what you often most "need" is a few less items in the closet so that you can make sense of what you have and evaluate it effectively.

Another problem with credit cards is that they often impel you to buy things you wouldn't actually purchase if you were paying cash. Credit cards are linked to instant gratification and impulse buying. If you insist on paying cash, you are more likely to consider your purchases for a long time before making them, to really weigh the pros and cons of a given item before bringing it into your home. You are also far less likely to accumulate faster than you can purge, because a credit line is often larger than a ready cash supply. Limited resources can keep us from buying things that aren't really needed.

Debt and Despair

The final problem with credit card purchases is directly related to a more emotional dimension of these purchases—debt. Americans are accumulating record amounts of debt at breakneck speed, perhaps because of the overabundance of great credit card offers. Credit card companies love to target college students, because they know that college students are notoriously poor and unrealistic. If these companies can "help" college students to spend money that they don't yet have, they can be assured of monthly payments, and better yet, they can freely raise APR rates when those payments don't come in on time.

These companies can also train young people to live by a debt mentality, so that even if they can get out of debt at certain phases of life, they will inevitably fall back into debt when the lure of certain items becomes too much for them. If you train people to buy more than they can afford—or to live by "soft," unrealistic numbers instead of limited resources—you can keep them in a continual position of dependency.

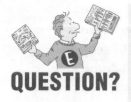

QUESTION?

Should I consolidate my balances with one of those low-interest credit cards?
Beware of credit card offers that offer a six-month low APR. Any credit card company that promises a temporary low rate may be planning to raise that rate to a much higher level after they've gotten you hooked. They are also free to raise your rate any time you miss a payment. This steady drain on your finances will cost you in the long run.

Ideally, before you make a credit card purchase, consider the emotional and economical costs of the purchase. Ask yourself how you will *feel* after you purchase the item, after you bring it home and begin to grapple with its real cost. This simple question can prevent purchases that may cause regret over the long haul.

Practice No-Net-Gain

In contemporary consumer society, many people struggle with excess. Even items you don't buy can come into your home. In Chicago and other cities, people leave household items that they no longer need in the back alley. The items could be as small as a toaster or as large as a sofa bed. Inevitably, within days a rattling truck comes down the alley, stopping at every dumpster to check and load.

These "salvage" trucks are usually loaded with an odd assortment of items—broken air conditioners, flat bike tires, children's books, and ratty sweaters. The mishmash is often tied together with a gigantic bungee cord. What ultimately becomes of this odd assortment is an urban mystery.

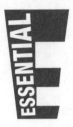

The FlyLady recommends: "Every time you buy something new, take the bag or bags they came in and pack up a similar item to give away. A born-organized friend of mine taught me this. I watched her add a new pair of tennis shoes to her closet and cull out an old pair for trash or charity."

Whenever you feel tempted to hold on to broken, useless items, or to bring in items that you don't really need, think of these trucks with their odd assortment of items. Imagine the task of sorting through these ever-growing piles, trying to cull value from heaps of junk. This task drains energy and time, resources that could be better spent managing those things that you already own.

Keep It Moving

The key to keeping clutter out of your home is to recognize that no matter what you do, clutter is a fact of life. It may come through a slow trickle of baby gifts, six bottles of shampoo that didn't quite work, or an assorted collection of spices that have lost their zing—or were never a good fit for your cooking habits in the first place. Perhaps you thought you loved Creole cooking, for example, and bought several spices only to find that you were never in the mood for that type of cuisine.

You might even have (as so many people do) broken appliances, such as washers and dryers, that no longer work—down in your basement, waiting for somebody to finally lug them off.

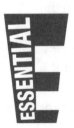

Some people seek to get rid of one item every single day. The item could be as small as a broken videotape, or as large as a saggy mattress. Over the course of a year, your home will have 365 fewer items, leaving you more room to live and grow into your space.

Although you might be able to remove 365 items this year, you may find that you will actually take in at least that much. Your attempts to simplify can become frustrated by the incredible amount of stuff that you will actively (or passively) bring into your home.

Counting Consumerism

Try counting items as they come in. If you have a small child who enjoys counting, get her involved in this educational exercise. Each time an item comes through the door, add it to your tally. At the end of each month, check to see how many items (books, clothes, personal products) came in. This will give you some idea of what you're up against.

Purging may be especially useful during significant changes in your life, when you know that you will either inevitably acquire more items than you can manage or need fewer items to make the present manageable. If you are about to move, now is a great time to start hauling things away, as every useless item you hang on to will inevitably cost you precious time, resources, energy, and money later on (learn more about planning a move in Chapter 19).

Create a Standard

You might like the idea of practicing no-net-gain, but you might feel unsure of how to begin. There are a few tried and true techniques that might be helpful as you seek to gain control of any clutter situation.

The first tip comes from the FlyLady. She recommends getting rid of the same type of item each time you bring a new item into your home. In practical terms, this means that if you purchase a new sweater, you should dig through your closet and find a ratty old sweater that you no longer wear or like. When you buy a new set of sneakers, dump the withered old pair in the trash.

Another useful way of sorting through household items is to create a standard by which you judge the things you have. This can be one of the most difficult things to do, because material possessions often have emotions attached to them. These attachments can obscure the real value (or lack thereof) in an object.

Scrutinize the items in your home—are they all functional, beautiful, helpful? If their function seems to be to gather dust, then it is time to find a new home for that object. If the item was once useful but is no longer useful, allow yourself to let it go, knowing that you will never regret living in a clutter-free environment. Trust that what goes around does come around. You can freely let items go, knowing that more items will inevitably find their way into your home.

Create a Clutter Out Box

The famed artist Andy Warhol had an unusual technique for managing clutter. He kept an empty cardboard box beside his desk, and when the clutter got to be too much for him, he simply tossed items into the box, taped it shut and then instructed an assistant to ship the box to New Jersey.

A display of these 612 cardboard boxes, called the *Time Capsules*, features a surprising variety of items—everything from insect-infested pizza dough to a palette used by Salvador Dali to letters from Mick Jagger. The most significant items are mixed in with irrelevant receipts and scraps from his life as a famous artist. One might have expected him to throw away the useless items and carefully put away the more valuable ones, but Warhol didn't seem to have the time or the inclination to sift through his things and separate the wheat from the chaff.

Managing Clutter

The contents of Warhol's *Time Capsules* can be viewed online at *www.warhol.org/tc21*. These cardboard boxes are fascinating, but not necessarily inspirational. Like Warhol, instead of actually organizing and purging, many people are tempted to just find increasingly inventive ways to store items. Within your own home, you may think you're "managing" clutter when in reality you're just moving it from one area to another. According to the Flylady, the goal is not to rearrange clutter, but to get it out the door.

It might be tempting to rent storage for items that don't fit in your home. While storage is sometimes helpful and necessary, in other situations it might prove to be a burden. Rented storage generates monthly bills and possible headaches and can delay decisions that are ultimately inevitable.

The Burden of Storage

When you feel tempted to rent storage, keep in mind that you will eventually be forced to contend with all those things that you store. This could mean renting a U-Haul truck and begging friends to help you to move the items. It could mean losing these items you've paid to store for years to flood, fire, or insects. Storage is often billed as a solution, but you do well to keep in mind that in many situations, storage just adds additional complexity.

You Can't Organize Clutter

There is one point that many home organizers can agree upon. Clutter, by its very definition, cannot be organized. While heroic efforts may temporarily make piles look orderly, the problem remains. The very amount of possessions in your home can sabotage your desire and will to clean.

The best alternative to storage is simplification. Instead of seeking more and more ways to hold on to more and more things, people can be better served by making decisions up-front. Instead of delaying the inevitable by tossing random items into a box and stuffing that box in a closet or attic, one can choose to create a "clutter out box."

Creating a clutter out box can be incredibly simple. A simple cardboard box (in the spirit of Andy Warhol) left by the back door can serve as a reminder to continually think in terms of purging. As soon you find that you're not using certain items, toss them in the box.

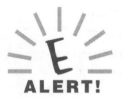

Certain items do belong in the trash. Stained shirts, pants with broken zippers, and shoes with floppy soles will not be seen as charitable gifts to those at the Salvation Army. Many charitable organizations also reject used baby items such as carseats, cribs, and highchairs because of liability and safety issues.

When the box is full, the FlyLady recommends that you bring it out to your car and place it in your trunk. That way, you don't really have to think about the task. You can just empty the box when you are running other errands, with a quick stop at the Salvation Army or any other business that takes used household items.

By starting small and trying to be consistent in the little things, you can reduce your debt, your stress, and your clutter. By cutting your tasks down to size, you keep them in the realm of the possible. Remember: If a journey of a thousand miles begins with a single step, then your job is just to start walking. Don't worry about how quickly or smoothly you'll complete the journey; just put one foot in front of the other and keep moving.

Chapter 5

The Home Office

While some people base their full-time careers in their homes, others simply need a space to keep records, bills, and related paperwork in order. Whatever your needs are, you can expect that these areas of your home will attract clutter and chaos. This chapter will offer advice on how to create and maintain an orderly home office. A comfortable, functional home office can increase your productivity and your impetus to get things done. This chapter will explore a variety of home-office spaces, as well as offering practical tips for keeping your office in order.

What Are Your Needs?

Before you begin to design and organize your home-office environment, create a detailed list of the types of work you'll be doing there. Keep in mind that you'll want to create a space where you'll want to be. For example, will the work require silence or should your office be located near the front door because of work-related visitors?

Those who work from home (and even those who simply pay bills and sort records there) know that it can be hard enough to motivate yourself to meet your goals. Don't add an extra reason to dread your job by placing your office in a dingy basement. Or if your job requires silence, don't place your desk in a household hub.

After you determine what tasks you hope to accomplish on an ongoing basis in the home office, develop a detailed list of furniture, equipment, and supplies required to achieve your objective. As you determine what's needed, think about ways you can reduce clutter in your workspace. For example, select furniture with plenty of drawers and filing cabinets with extra storage space. You should also position equipment close to electrical outlets and phone jacks, so you won't have lots of unsightly and disorganized cords running throughout the room.

Because your desk is the central and most integral part of your home office, decide on its location first. Then determine what other furniture and equipment needs to be nearby and what can be placed elsewhere in the room. This will help you create the most functional design and layout for your work environment.

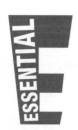

Julie Morgenstern suggests that if you generate your income through a variety of different types of home-based work, think in terms of creating activity hubs within your office. That way, you'll be better able to assign "homes" to the items associated with your different jobs, and you'll also increase your productivity by "visiting" each area daily.

Once you have a basic idea of what you hope to accomplish in your home workspace and what equipment you'll need in order to achieve your objectives, design and lay out your home office so that it will maximize your productivity and be a comfortable place to work. Issues such as lighting, color schemes, ergonomics, and functionality all need to be addressed. As with any organizational task, planning is crucial, so put some thought into your needs and wants, and then address each issue individually.

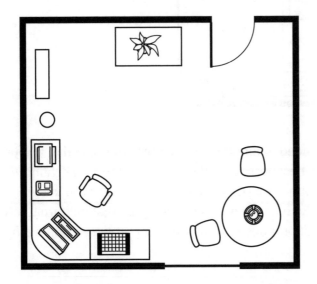

A typical office arrangement.

Before making a major financial investment in remodeling an area of your home to transform it into a home office, try working in the area for a while to ensure that the environment and surroundings will help you maximize your productivity. Certain problems, such as noise, traffic, or lack of natural light, could remain even if you remodel, so take care to select an area that you like being in.

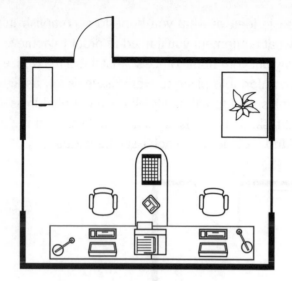

A home office with
an L-shaped desk for
more workspace.

Remember, you need to pinpoint an area of your home that will provide ample space and the best possible environment (in terms of lighting, temperature, privacy, and sound) for you to be productive. After you know what furniture you'll need, take measurements to make sure that the furniture you're planning to use will fit properly in your current or proposed home office.

Lighting Your Office

In addition to having a place that's quiet, you want it to be properly lighted. Ideally, a home office will have at least one large window and/or skylight to allow natural daylight into the room. The lamps, lighting fixtures, and light bulbs you choose will also impact the overall environment. For example, fluorescent light bulbs may be cheaper and last longer, but they're much tougher on your eyes (and your mood) than traditional light bulbs. Plus, part of the luxury of working from home is that you can be productive without being forced to function in an industrial environment—seize the freedom you have and make your office ideally suited to your own needs.

Studies have shown that people exposed to natural sunlight tend to be happier and more productive in a work environment. Natural sunlight can be supplemented by full-spectrum light bulbs that simulate natural sunlight. Others, however, feel that a view distracts them from their work. The novelist

Kent Haruf, for example, pens his novels in an old coal room in his basement, and he likes to type his first draft with his eyes closed.

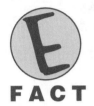

FACT

Many paper items can be tossed or recycled. You usually don't need to hold on to early drafts of reports or proposals. Likewise, most magazines now have online databases with easy-to-use search boxes. Recycle any magazine if you know that you can also find the articles online.

Choosing Your Desk and Storage Supplies

The most important piece of furniture in any home office is the desk. You want your desk to be functional and comfortable, just the right height so that you don't have to hunch over it, and with enough space to spread out your papers.

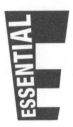

Important documents such as birth certificates, marriage certificates, passports, adoption paperwork, and divorce papers should be stored in a fireproof lockbox or in a safety deposit box. Make sure you have photocopies of all these documents on hand, but that the originals are stored in an extremely secure location.

As you choose a desk, consider U-shaped or L-shaped designs that provide ample space for a computer, lamp, papers, telephone, etc., but also give you space to do your work. If you incorporate a computer desk into your home office, make sure it's ergonomically designed. The ideal height of the keyboard should be about twenty-eight inches, yet the monitor should be at eye level so that you're not looking up or down at it.

The desk design you ultimately choose should be based upon what you'll be using the desk for. For example, if you'll be holding business meetings around your desk, you'll need ample room for chairs on both sides of the desk, plus a clear line of sight to the people sitting opposite you.

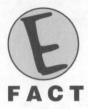

FACT

If you have bulky supplies in your office that you use rarely, perhaps you should move them into accessible storage. For printers, scanners, and other electronic equipment, purchase a cabinet where you can tuck these items away—just be sure that your storage cabinet has decent ventilation, as electrical items do need air to circulate around them.

For most people, desk space is a priority. Thus, you want to have at your disposal as much open desk space as possible, based on the amount of room in your home office. Take measurements and create your own blueprint on paper. This will allow you to experiment with different room designs so you can have the largest desk possible, yet not feel as if this piece of furniture dominates the room or makes for a claustrophobic workspace. Most home organizers recommend that you position your desk first and then arrange other pieces of furniture around it.

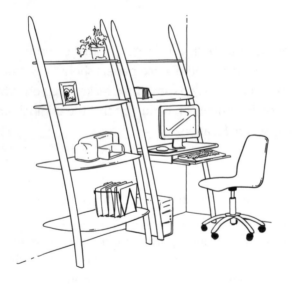

A creative office desk saves space.

Focus on the Essentials

Keep in mind that you'll probably want important files, your computer (and printer), telephone, calculator, and/or other items within arm's reach in order to maximize your productivity. To ensure that what you need is readily available, get rid of nonessential furniture and other items. Many physical items that used to take up precious desk space can now be found on your computer—you won't need a calculator or calendar if these items are available on your computer.

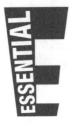

As soon as you complete a project, take a few moments to return all books, articles, and tools to their proper homes. As you put these items away, you communicate to yourself that you have eliminated one more project from your to-do list and that you now have the space to move on to fresh projects.

Likewise, while you'll want your computer printer within arm's reach so that you don't have to leave your chair to obtain a printout, your fax machine can probably be placed farther away and not stored on your main desk.

Creative Storage

Be sure to utilize the available space to its greatest potential. For example, instead of having file bins on your desk, can you utilize hanging files and take advantage of nearby wall space? A computer-monitor stand with a shelf above and a drawer underneath it is also an excellent tool for saving valuable desk space. This type of stand will ensure that your computer monitor will be at eye level, and thus inflict less stress on your neck, shoulders, and arms.

Office supplies, shipping supplies, and other items should be readily available. Consider purchasing drawer organizers to keep your office tools compartmentalized. For bulky items like industry magazines and articles, consider dual-function furniture—perhaps you can store these inside an ottoman with a pull-off top.

The Great Paper Chase

Many people struggle with paper clutter in their offices. One of the best ways to keep paper at bay is to not let it through the door. Unread newspapers and magazines should be recycled quickly. Don't burden yourself with guilt simply because you don't have time to read them. Marla Cilley, the FlyLady, takes her magazines to the dentist, doctor, and mechanic and leaves them there on a coffee table. By doing this, she declutters her own home while offering something potentially useful to these waiting rooms.

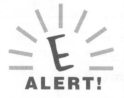

ALERT!

Medical and dental records should be kept in a separate file box. Immunization records are especially important and could be needed even when your children start college. Don't count on your doctor to store these records for you, because she can purge or lose these items over time.

Creating an In Box/Out Box

You can also utilize an in box/out box or a to-do box. All papers, except the ones you're currently working with, should be placed within one of these boxes, properly filed in a filing cabinet, or thrown away. Don't allow yourself to create piles of papers, reports, bills, mail, and other documents on the floor or on nearby chairs. After these piles grow, they become more and more daunting and require more and more time to organize.

Office supplies and tools you use regularly—such as your stapler, tape, paper clips, rubber bands, pens, pencils, memo pads and notepads, staple remover, markers, scissors, rulers, and so on—should be kept in a desk drawer that's readily available and within arm's reach. These items should not clutter your desktop when they're not in use. Also, purge supply drawers frequently so that you know exactly what you have and what you need. You don't want to keep a client on hold while you try to hunt down a working pen.

To make your drawers more functional, purchase dividers that create small pockets for each of your supplies. This will help you to keep your drawers in order and to quickly locate everything you need.

Keeping your office free of clutter will require a certain amount of consistency on your part, but it can be done. You only need to feel the rewards of having an orderly office to find the motivation to keep it that way.

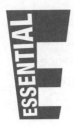

On a regular basis, sort through your desk drawers and throw away dead pens, bent paper clips, stretched-out rubber bands, and other useless junk that has accumulated. Don't save business cards if you can index contacts on your computer more efficiently.

Home-Office Seating

At the end of a workday, does your lower back hurt or do you feel tension in your neck and shoulders? These pains may be caused by your office chair and could be reduced or eliminated if you purchase an ergonomically designed chair that better fits your body.

Chairs are one of the most important home-office tools, yet they tend to be overlooked. An ergonomically designed office chair may cost a bit more than a traditional chair, but they're designed to support the contours and movements of your body. Ergonomic chairs are also adjustable to meet your unique needs based on your height, weight, posture, and work habits.

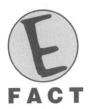

FACT

Although it might be expensive to invest in a top-quality chair, think of this purchase as an investment in your long-term health and your career. Uncomfortable chairs will increase exhaustion and can lead to chronic pain. If cost is an issue, go for a top-quality chair but buy it used.

Optimally, the chair should also offer some sort of lumbar adjustment, because everyone has a different spinal alignment that needs to be considered. Additionally, these chairs should have rounded edges with adjustable arms. If you're typing at a keyboard and using a mouse, your arms will be in a different position than if you're simply doing paperwork at your desk. A chair also needs to be moveable, so it should be on wheels and have swivel capability.

Studies show that people who use ergonomically designed chairs are more productive, because they're more comfortable throughout the day. Their bodies undergo less stress, and their lower bodies experience improved circulation. The price of a high-quality, well-designed ergonomic chair will typically range from $500 to $700, depending on its features.

Filing Cabinets

Filing cabinets come in a wide range of sizes. Use as much vertical space as possible by investing in a four-drawer vertical file cabinet. This takes up the least amount of actual floor space, yet can store the most papers. Your most time-sensitive and important papers can be kept directly on your desk using a desktop file holder. It's common for people to utilize an in box or to-do file directly on their desks. The trick, however, is to be disciplined enough to process those important papers promptly, so that they don't accumulate and become unmanageable.

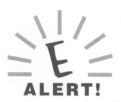

ALERT!

Avoid cheap filing cabinets. Filing cabinets need to be durable enough to endure years of use and the weight of your paperwork. Cheap filing cabinets come apart over time or become difficult to open and close. Reduce the temptation to put off filing by purchasing filing cabinets that are a joy to use.

Use separate file cabinets for your personal and business files. Next, divide up your files and label them carefully. For example, in your personal filing cabinet, you may have folders or separate files for the following types of paperwork: auto-related, banking, bills, career, education, financial, health/medical, insurance, investments, legal, mortgage, taxes (keeping current and past information separate), travel, and warranties/receipts/instructions.

All of your files should be divided up, labeled, and kept organized. Files can be sorted and stored alphabetically, numerically, with some sort of color-coding, by date, geographically, by subject, or by using your own criteria. Keep your filing system straightforward, up-to-date, and intuitive for others. For example, if you're storing company files, store them alphabetically by company name (or the client's last name).

Keep current files readily available, and keep dormant/inactive files in airtight storage containers in an out-of-the way area, such as a basement or attic. Old files can also be scanned into a computer and stored on a computer's hard drive or in an electronic format, which will save you space and eliminate clutter. An inexpensive document scanner can dramatically simplify this task.

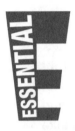

Set aside fifteen minutes a week to purge old files that you no longer need. In most cases, you don't need to save earlier drafts of proposals or projects. Check with your accountant to determine how frequently bills, cancelled checks, and tax records can be purged.

Dozens, perhaps hundreds of papers will cross your desk each day. For those papers that deserve your utmost attention, that can't be forgotten, or that you classify as having top priority, consider placing a special file on your desk or hanging a bulletin board near your desk upon which you can stick only the most important of papers.

Organizing Your Computer

By using off-the-shelf computer software in conjunction with a powerful operating system, you can perform a wide range of tasks and better organize the immense amount of information you receive. Because the cost of computers and related equipment continues to drop while the power and capabilities of computers increase, more and more people are relying on technology to handle a greater range of everyday tasks.

It's important that you, as the user, determine exactly the tasks you'll ultimately be using your computer for. No matter what applications you choose to utilize, think of the computer's hard drive (the place where your files, programs, and data are stored) as an electronic filing system that also needs to be kept organized.

However, simply by using your everyday programs, your computer generates random files that fill up your hard drive but that you don't need. For example, the Web browser Microsoft Explorer keeps track of every Web site you visit and stores detailed information about those sites in various cache and temporary folders and files. To delete some of the older Microsoft Explorer files that may no longer be needed, from the Tools drop-down menu in the program, select the Internet Options feature. You can then adjust the Temporary Internet Files settings or delete the unnecessary files.

Data Back-Up Options

You'll want to be sure that you back up all of your computer files. Backup files can be stored on writable CD-ROMs, Zip disks, or another form of data backup device.

It is critical to make regular backups of your work. Data loss can and does happen—your hard drive can become corrupt, a hurricane can take out your house (depending where you live), thieves may break in and steal your computer, a computer virus can wipe out your hard drive, or lightning can fry your electronics. Backups can be made to a Zip or Flash drive, an external hard drive, or over the Internet (through a service such as Strongspace or Rsync.net). Network backups can protect you even in the case of theft. Although keeping backups may take some time and cost some money, these costs pale in comparison to the risk of losing years of work.

Taming Cables

Have you looked behind your computer lately? If you're like most people who have a computer, monitor, printer, scanner, mouse, external speakers, and other devices connected to your computer, chances are you'll see a maze of wires tangled behind your desk. While you may not be able to create an entirely wire-free environment, you can sort through all of those wires one time, bind them together, label each of them, and ultimately create a more organized workspace.

Most office-supply stores sell Velcro strips for wrapping wires and making them neater. (Twist ties also work perfectly.) Many computer desks also offer special compartments and holes in the desktop for routing wires and keeping them out of open view.

Consider a Laptop

You may think laptop computers are only for students and people who travel for their jobs, but the truth is a laptop can be a valuable asset for just about anyone in any profession. With regard to home organization, laptops take up a lot less space on your desk, which means you have more room for other important materials. And because laptops are portable, you will always have the option of taking your computer into another room, to a coffee shop or library, or even on a plane. Laptops all have battery packs, so they can often run for several hours without being plugged in. Laptops tend to be more expensive than desktop computers, but the benefits of a small, lightweight, portable computer can easily outweigh the extra cost.

If you don't have enough in your budget for a new laptop, consider buying one used. You can look online (eBay, Amazon, craigslist, etc.), or just keep an eye out for local listings in the newspaper. An older laptop might not have a built-in video camera or DVD burner, but it can still get the job done.

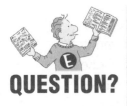

QUESTION?

My computer takes up so much space on the desk with all its components. Are there other neater options out there?
Yes! There are many different types of computers out there. For example, if you're looking to save valuable desk space, consider adding a flat-screen monitor to your computer. These monitors are often only several inches thick, yet offer excellent resolution. They're also easier on your eyes if you use your computer for extended periods of time.

Organizing Your Contacts and Information

One challenge virtually everyone faces is keeping track of all the people they know. Contacts grow—most people have home, work, and cell numbers, as well as Web sites and e-mail addresses.

You could try maintaining a handwritten address book, but each time information needs to be added or changed, keeping those handwritten pages neat and legible may become more and more of a challenge. Keeping a business-card file is also an option, but finding the right business card when you need it after your collection starts to grow can be a time-consuming task. In today's information-oriented world, using contact management software offers the ideal solution for keeping track of the people you know as well as other important data.

Maintaining Your Contact Database

After you've begun developing and maintaining your own contact database, people's phone numbers, addresses, and other information will be available to you almost instantly, as long as you're in front of your computer. By also utilizing a hand-held personal digital assistant (PDA) or other portable device (such as an iPod), you can take this important information with you wherever you go.

Choosing an Office Telephone

Your telephone is your primary connection with the outside world. Depending on the type of work you do, you may find it necessary to have multiple phone lines in your home office: a personal phone line, a work phone line, a modem line, and/or a fax line. Think about how many phone lines you'll need and what they'll be used for before purchasing your actual equipment.

When ordering voice phone service from the phone company, you'll be offered many options and service add ons. In addition to choosing which phone company will provide your local and long-distance phone service, you may be offered call waiting, call forwarding, three-way calling, caller ID, and an incoming toll-free number. Based on what you'll be using your phone for, you can choose the services that will help you be the most productive.

If you have a high-speed cable connection, a voice over Internet Protocol (VOIP) line can cut costs significantly, and may come with added benefits such as the ability to receive voice-mail messages through e-mail. On the downside, a VOIP line may not work in a power outage, may require rewiring to work through the house, and may require a little too much tech savvy. If you have DSL (a high-speed Internet connection through your phone line), a VOIP line may not save you much money, since many phone companies offer good bundled rates.

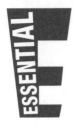

Caller ID is an invaluable resource for those who work from home. Sometimes, communicating to friends and family that your working hours are as valuable as those spent in an office can be a challenge. Caller ID will allow you to ignore personal calls and solicitations so that you can reduce distractions and increase your productivity.

In addition to the phone service you choose, you'll also need to purchase a telephone. As you'll quickly discover, you have many options available. Phones come in all shapes and sizes and have a wide range of features built into them. Many phones also offer features such as a built-in answering machine, caller ID, speed dialing, a hold button, a speakerphone, a mute button, a headset, and conference calling. Determine in advance which of these functions you want to utilize. If you want to use a wireless Internet connection, make sure your cordless phone is not 2.4 GHz, since this can interfere with wireless transmissions.

Telephone headsets are ideal if you want to talk on the phone but keep your hands free to use a computer keyboard, for example. If you'll regularly be making business calls, find a phone that doesn't allow background noise (such as children playing or dogs barking) to be heard.

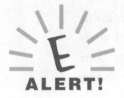

ALERT!

Although cordless phones are convenient, make sure you have at least one corded phone in your home. Should you lose power, cordless phones will not work because they require electricity. Also, if you will conduct taped or radio interviews from your office, invest in a high-quality corded phone that does not have a hum.

Plan for Productivity

After you've had an opportunity to bring some order to your home office, think about ways to organize your work habits. Try to establish work patterns for yourself. For example, after you create your to-do list each morning, allocate time to open your mail, deal with incoming e-mail, and do whatever other tasks are an important part of your routine. As you plan your day, schedule some flexible time to manage unexpected distractions and problems.

The National Association of Professional Organizers (NAPO) is a not-for-profit professional association whose members include organizational consultants, speakers, trainers, authors, and manufacturers of organizing products. NAPO's mission is to encourage the development of professional organizers and promote the recognition and advancement of the professional-organizing industry.

Implementing an organizational system can help you deal with everything from your papers to your professional responsibilities and give you parameters on what to keep, what to toss, and what to take action on.

NAPO offers these suggestions for increased productivity and organization on their Web site at *www.napo.net*:

- Break large projects down into small, sequential steps, and then schedule these steps into your day using your personal planner, scheduler, or PDA.
- Keep only the supplies you need daily on your desktop.

- Be clear about the response you need when sending a message (voice mail, e-mail, or a letter) to a colleague. They can then provide a full response, even if they don't reach you directly.
- Keep a file index (a master list of file names). Check the index before creating a new file to avoid making duplicates, and use it when deciding where to file a piece of paper.

After you've had an opportunity to tackle the clutter and to bring the tools you need into your office, you might find that you actually have to work less, and yet your productivity naturally increases. When you don't have to chase down paperwork or dig for contact information, small tasks can be done swiftly and you'll have more energy and time to devote to the more essential and lucrative tasks.

Chapter 6

Organizing the Kitchen

The kitchen may be the heart of the home, but it is also the place that naturally attracts the most clutter and chaos. The combination of such a wide variety of items that need to be stored and the high traffic can make this room especially challenging. This chapter will explore a variety of ways to organize your kitchen, transforming it into a place of beauty, order, and simplicity, where you and your family will want to gather, cook, and linger.

Clutter-Free Countertops

In every area of home organization, begin with the basics. Kitchen counters often attract clutter, and this can lead to a crowded, defeated look. Go into your kitchen and assess the items on your counters. Do all of them need to be there? Are there some small appliances on your counters that you don't use daily (or use very rarely)? Consider finding a new home for these appliances—either tuck them away in a cabinet or give them to someone who will use them.

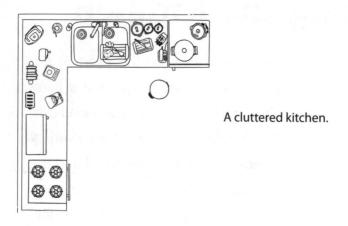

A cluttered kitchen.

To free-up counter space, use appliances (such as a microwave) that can be installed under your cabinets. Also, can you install a telephone on a nearby wall with an extra-long handset cord (or a cordless handset), so that you can travel around the entire kitchen area unimpeded by cords? Can you utilize a paper-towel rack that hangs on a wall or on the side of your refrigerator so that it doesn't take up countertop space?

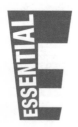

Marla Cilley recommends that you strive to empty your dishwasher immediately after the cycle is complete. This way, you'll reduce sink clutter (no dirty dishes will get trapped in a "holding pattern") and, if your family members know that the dishwasher won't be full of clean dishes for hours on end, they'll be easier to train to fill it.

If you do your dishes by hand, beware of the dish rack. Not only can it be tempting to let dishes pile up there, but the moisture can create an ideal climate for mold and bacteria to grow (unwelcome creatures such as roaches love this kind of dank environment). You might want to buy a stainless steel rack or any rack that is easy to clean and attractive. If you begin with an attractive rack, you'll feel more inclined to keep it looking nice— you'll be better able to see it as well, when you keep those dishes moving!

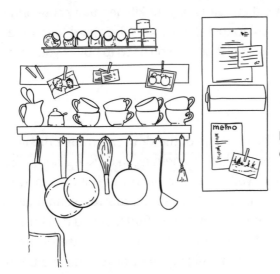

Keep your counters clear by optimizing wall space.

Cabinets and Drawers

For some people, the idea of tackling those kitchen cabinets and drawers can be almost paralyzing. There is just so much to do and it can be hard to know where to start. Keep in mind that you don't have to do it all at once— in fact, you probably shouldn't even try, because you might crash and burn. Instead, take it one drawer and one cabinet at a time. If you can do one cabinet or drawer each day for a couple of weeks, you'll find that this small amount of daily effort will radically change the way your kitchen looks and feels.

One Drawer at a Time

To begin with, take a single drawer and dump out the contents. The incredible variety of items might even make you laugh—that's good! Enjoy learning about yourself and your own quirky habits as you organize.

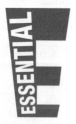

As you organize your kitchen, focus first on the areas that have been creating headaches. Are there parts of your kitchen that cause annoying delays every time you go there? Are your spices hard to reach and are you never quite certain which spices you need to buy or you already own? Start there.

After you've emptied the contents of the drawer, arrange the items into three piles. These piles can be titled something like "Keep here," "Store in another place," and "Goodbye." As you reduce the bulk in each drawer, you'll find that it will be much easier to keep the drawer clean. Plus, it feels great to open a formerly cluttered drawer and find that you can immediately spot the items you need—the boost in efficiency and ease of use will be well worth your efforts. Just try organizing one drawer and see if it doesn't make you want to do more!

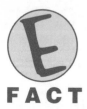

FACT

A huge variety of drawer and cupboard sorters are available. Two of them might be especially worthwhile additions to your kitchen—a silverware sorter and, for the cupboards, the "step shelves" for cans and spices. If your cans are more visible you will save money, because you won't be tempted to replace items you already own.

As you sort through your cabinets and drawers, think in terms of categories. Some entire categories of items might be able to go in another room—fine linens and china, for example, might find a place in your dining room.

Special items for entertaining can also be located together so that you'll have quick access to them when company arrives.

After your kitchen items are divided into categories, determine whether each group needs cabinet space, drawer space, or some other type of storage. Will all of these items be kept in the kitchen, or will some items, such as your fine china, be kept in the formal dining area? Measure all of your available cabinet space and make sure that the items you plan to store there will fit.

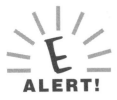

ALERT!

Arrange your cupboards so that things used most frequently are in the easiest-to-reach places. Organize the pantry so that breakfast cereals, beverages, and other packaged foods are easy to locate. With spices, create a system that works for you—for instance, you can group spices as "baking spices," "cooking spices," and "ethnic spices."

By arranging your food in an accessible and easy-to-spot way, you'll find that cooking is simpler. You'll also be far less likely to be confused about what you do and don't need come grocery day, and you'll save money as a result.

Special-Care Items

Keep in mind that certain items will need special care to keep them from becoming dull or damaged. A hardwood knife block (stored on a countertop) or a magnetic wall-mounted knife rack/utensil holder may be more suitable than a drawer for your fancy knives and cutlery.

Spices do lose their zest over time and should be replaced when this occurs. Keep in mind, however, that the conventional wisdom that spices should be replaced every three to six months may not be correct. Specialty-spice companies recommend that you keep your spices as long as they have flavor—in some cases, they can last years. Just be sure to store them in airtight containers, away from heat and direct sunlight.

An Orderly Fridge and Freezer

The first step in organizing your refrigerator and freezer is to empty it out and clean it. Remove all of the shelves and clean them. If you have glass or plastic shelves, try using a natural cleaner without harmful chemicals. Because the refrigerator is a contained and well-sealed space, you don't want chemicals compromising the indoor air quality—or leaving residue on your apples and blueberries.

Start on the top shelf. Decide what will be kept, and then throw away old leftovers—let go of items that you know you'll never eat. Open all containers and check what's inside. Throw out anything that's out of date or questionable.

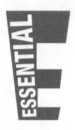

If you find that fruits and veggies often languish in your refrigerator, place them at eye level so that the moment you open the door you'll be enticed to eat or prepare them. An overstuffed refrigerator can also contribute to this problem. Clear out leftovers quickly so you can easily view and assess the contents of your fridge.

Next, inventory the items that belong in your refrigerator and decide how you'll organize them. Take full advantage of the drawers, shelves, and refrigerator door. Keep similar items together. Store small, loose items and leftovers in clear-plastic containers so you can see what's inside.

Never keep eggs in the refrigerator door. This will expose them to air each time the door is opened and closed. Instead, keep them in the carton on an upper shelf in the refrigerator.

Crisper drawers are good for vegetables, such as peppers. These drawers typically have humidity controls designed to help prevent vegetables from losing moisture. (The drawers seal tightly, which limits oxygen intake. The more oxygen intake, the quicker a food will deteriorate and spoil.)

Keep lettuce fresher by storing it unwashed in a heavy-duty zipper bag. Discard the outer leaves that contain excess moisture. Wrap the lettuce in a paper towel, insert it in the plastic bag, squeeze as much air out of the bag as possible, and seal the bag.

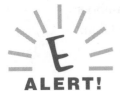

When it comes to meat, "When in doubt, throw it out." It is better to waste a little beef than to suffer food poisoning. Fresh fish should be consumed within a few days.

Items for the Freezer

If you wish to store fresh herbs such as basil, store them in the freezer door in a plastic bag. In addition, store whole-wheat flour in the freezer. (White flour, however, can be stored at room temperature.) Freeze meats that you don't plan to use within three days. Store items in airtight containers, such as freezer bags and Tupperware. Make sure you date all items. Most frozen items, such as soups, casseroles and meat, can keep for several months in the freezer. Just be sure that oxygen doesn't get in and cause freezer burn, which will compromise flavor.

Room-Temperature Items

Though you may be tempted to put all fresh foods in the fridge, this isn't a good idea for certain foods. For example, don't store potatoes in the refrigerator. The starch breaks down quickly, which leaves the potato mushy if baked. In the same way, tomatoes and cucumbers should be stored at room temperature. If you want these items cold in a salad, chill them before serving. Bananas, avocados, and zucchini should also be kept out.

Avoiding Bacterial Contamination

Not only is keeping your kitchen clean an absolute must for maintaining an organized environment, it's also critical for maintaining your health. If the kitchen is not kept clean, bacteria and mold can grow on the surfaces and get into your food, which could result in serious illness. Whether you're storing perishable foods, cooking, or cleaning, there are all kinds of safety measures you should take within your kitchen.

The Partnership for Food Safety Education sponsors the Fight Bac! Web site (*www.fightbac.org*), which offers an abundance of information about keeping your food safe from dangerous bacteria. It recommends taking these four primary precautions:

Clean: Wash hands and surfaces often
Separate: Don't cross-contaminate!
Cook: Cook to proper temperature
Chill: Refrigerate promptly

Avoid Cross-Contamination

When working in the kitchen, wash your hands, utensils, and kitchen surfaces often. After a knife or plate touches raw meat, wash it immediately. Wash your hands, using warm and soapy water, before and after you handle raw foods. Wash your cutting board, dishes, utensils, and countertops after each use (especially after preparing raw meat, poultry, or fish). Use separate cutting boards for raw meats and vegetables.

Store meats, poultry, and fish away from other foods. Wrap or package each separately. Ask your local butcher for information on how to properly store specific types of meat, fish, and poultry for short (one to three days) or long periods of time.

Managing Coupons

How would you like to save $5, $10, or even $50 every time you shop at the supermarket? If this sounds appealing, coupon clipping may be the answer. Searching for and clipping coupons from the newspaper or from advertising circulars can be a time-consuming task, but many people find this to be a relaxing rainy-day or Sunday-afternoon activity.

You can use a binder with clear pockets to sort, categorize, and store your coupons. For example, you may have categories called "Cleaning Products" and "Pet Care Products," and you simply place all related coupons in that category within the same pocket.

An alternative is to use a small file box and store your coupons alphabetically, either by product name or brand name. For example, Ivory soap could be filed under "I" for Ivory or "S" for soap, depending on your coupon filing system.

Another alternative is to use a batch of small envelopes, each marked with a separate coupon category. All the envelopes can be stored together in a larger one so that they are kept together.

Storing Coupons

Using coupons can be a fun way to save money, if you're willing to invest the time needed to clip the coupons, bring them to the store, find the right product, and redeem the coupon. As a general rule, clip and store coupons for only those products you already use (or definitely want to try). If you're not careful, your coupon file could easily get cluttered with coupons you have no intention of using.

Before you cut out a coupon, pay attention to the expiration date and the fine print. Also before clipping it, determine what exactly you need to purchase to redeem the coupon. If you're required to purchase an extra-large container of laundry detergent but you need only a small container, do the math and find out how much the savings will be if you purchase the larger container using the coupon.

After you clip your coupons, create a written shopping list for yourself. On the list, place a star or some other notation next to the items you have a coupon for. Next to that item, list the specific name brand and size you need to purchase in order to redeem the coupon.

So, where can the best coupons be found? For starters, try the Sunday newspaper and look for inserts and circulars. Look also in the newspaper's weekly food section, which typically appears on Wednesdays. You can also find coupons in general-interest magazines and in women's magazines.

Coupon Swap

Many supermarkets and libraries offer coupon swap-boxes for consumers. Drop off your unused coupons and grab a few you'll actually use in order to save money. Many supermarkets also have in-store displays that dispense coupons that you can use at checkout.

Before you shop, visit the Web site of the supermarket where you typi-cally shop. Online coupons (which you can print out and redeem) may be offered. There are also Web sites dedicated specifically to distributing cou-pons to consumers online. Check out the following:

- *www.centsoff.com*
- *www.ecoupons.com*
- *www.refundsweepers.com/foodstores.shtml*
- *www.smartsource.net*

Organizing Recipes

If you enjoy cooking, chances are, over time you'll acquire many recipes in many different forms—from cookbooks and magazine clippings to print-outs from the Internet and handwritten notes from friends and family. One way of storing these recipes is to purchase a three-ring binder with dividers, along with a handful of clear protective sheets that you can insert papers into. Divide the binder up into sections, such as "Appetizers," "Desserts," "Chicken Dishes," and so on, and then file your recipes within the binder. Keep this binder with your cookbooks, on a shelf in the kitchen.

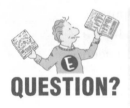

QUESTION?

My cookbooks always get all dirty and covered in food when I have them out on the counter. Is there any way to prevent this?
Invest in a cookbook holder with a protective shield. These products come in various styles and sizes, and they hold your cookbook open to the page you're referring to while protecting the pages. Most are small enough or collapsible for easy storage.

An alternative is to file your recipes in a file cabinet or even on the com-puter. You can find several off-the-shelf electronic-cookbook computer-software packages on the market. In addition, you can use a database management program to enter and file your own recipes. You can also use your PDA to create and maintain your grocery-shopping list. Because a PDA is totally portable, you can carry it around throughout the day and take it to the supermarket.

Trash and Recyclables

What goes in must come out. This is especially the case with the kitchen, where you bring a huge amount of food, packaging, and other containers in, and many of these things will need to eventually be disposed of. Have you ever read Shel Silverstein's poem "Sarah Cynthia Sylvia Stout Would Not Take the Garbage Out"? This kind of stench and disarray can come if you don't have a good system for managing garbage and recyclables.

Choosing a Garbage Can

Garbage cans with lids are ideal for keeping bad smells in and pets out. Stainless steel can also be attractive and can endure for many years. If you purchase a can that uses a foot lever, you'll reduce the risk of picking up bacteria while cooking. After your garbage bag is full, seal and dispose of it as quickly as possible. If you're tossing food scraps, place these scraps within a small plastic bag that can be sealed and toss that into the larger garbage bag. This will reduce bad odors.

To maintain a clean environment, you'll also want to spray your garbage can with disinfectant spray (that also removes odor) and clean the garbage can itself on a regular basis.

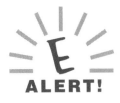

ALERT!

Your garbage should not be accessible to pets or children. If you must spend more to purchase a garbage can with a lid that can be opened only by foot, this investment will pay off. Visits to the vet are costly, and certain items, such as plastic, chocolate, or corncobs, can endanger your pet's life.

Compost

If you're a gardener, you know that food scraps can have a second life as compost. Decomposed food scraps can provide rich nutrients to your soil. Instead of scraping off your plates into the trash can or garbage disposal, put fruit and vegetable scraps into an airtight jug. As these items slowly decompose, you can add them to your soil for the health of your plants.

You can buy small, discreet countertop compost pails at many home stores. These items make it easy to gather peels, eggshells, and other food-waste indoors, while keeping odors to a minimum. You can store a compost pail under the sink, on the counter, or in a cabinet for accessibility.

Managing Recyclables

Recycling is a great way to reduce waste and to conserve resources. Most American cities now have dynamic recycling programs. Minimal effort is required on your part to make recycling work in your home.

First of all, make sure that you rinse all cans and glass bottles well. These bottles, cans, and boxes can stink and attract pests if they are left with residue on them. In most cities, you will be expected to foot-flatten food cartons and plastic bottles and jugs. You'll also be expected to separate green, brown, blue, and clear glass as well as newspapers and cereal boxes.

If you purchase a recycling sorter with at least two separate bins, this can simplify your task. Keep in mind, however, that, like trash, even well-rinsed bottles and cans will create a sticky, stinky residue in your bin. The bin will need to be washed frequently.

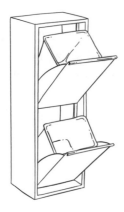

Simplify recycling with a double bin.

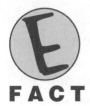

In most cities, you don't need to remove labels from your cans because the high temperature used for processing recyclables can easily remove them. You do, however, want to remove lids, which are not reused and can be a nuisance for your recycling company.

Ideally, you'll take your recycling out as quickly as possible. If you live in an area where you keep large color-coded bins out back at all times, you can simply store your recycling in plastic grocery bags and then carry them out each morning or evening. This is especially the case with newspapers—they tend to create a lot of clutter and can be cumbersome, if you try to take out too many at the same time. Just as you bring in a single newspaper each morning, try to take out (or place in a recycling container) a single newspaper each night. By tackling your recycling quickly, you can prevent the work and mess involved in managing a larger recycling system.

Creating a Family Message Center

If you live in a household with other people, chances are you all have very different schedules—and it can be hard to coordinate all these schedules. You might want to create a family message center in the kitchen. This message center may include a large corkboard or dry-erase board for posting messages and bins for sorting each individual's mail. On the message board, you can maintain a food-shopping list that all members of the family can contribute to.

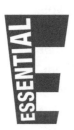

Stores like Target, Staples, and the Container Store carry lots of great products you can use to create a family message center—from dry-erase boards and bulletin boards to baskets and filing trays. By buying individual pieces at one of these stores, you can customize your family message center to accommodate your family's unique needs.

A family message center can help ease stress that comes from miscommunication, because there will be a common place for messages to be left. Everyone in the family will know to check the message board so that even when schedules conflict, family members can communicate about upcoming events and household chores. You can also use the message board to leave kind words for those you live with. A little bit of kindness can go a long way to ease tensions and bring harmony.

Love Your Kitchen

This chapter has dealt primarily with the nuts and bolts of organizing your kitchen, but sheer organization won't make you love the space (although it can certainly help!). But there are a few things you can do that are inexpensive and go a long way toward making your kitchen a place where you'll want to be. American people tend to eat out almost 50 percent of the time. This high rate is related to many different factors—demanding work schedules, general fatigue, and a desire to have somebody else wash up at the end of a long day.

This high number of meals eaten out of the home tends to harm our bodies and possibly even our souls. At a restaurant, you might be tempted to overeat because of the large portion sizes. Also, meals out are often noisy and busy. They don't tend to give people the downtime they might really need at the end of the day. If you can learn to love being in your kitchen, you might find that you are less inclined to want to eat elsewhere.

Buy Your Groceries in a Store You Love

Victoria Moran, in her book *Shelter for the Spirit*, recommends that you shop for your groceries in a store you would want to go to even if you didn't need to buy food. If you bring home foods that you love from a store that you love, you will be more likely to want to stay home and consume them. Victoria Moran writes, "Wherever you choose to shop, remember that every time you bring a bag of groceries into your house or apartment, you are bringing something of the store in with them. How do you want your house to feel? Shop in places that feel that way, too."

Many cities have wonderful farmers' markets that provide local, seasonal fare. By supporting local farmers, you're able to eat food that you can trust. Because the produce is so fresh, it often looks like edible art. You can make the most of your fresh items from the farmers' market by displaying veggies in a large bowl on your table—this functional centerpiece can be as lovely as it is useful.

When you organize your refrigerator, don't just think in terms of making it functional. Think in terms of beauty as well. Fresh produce can be placed in attractive bowls in your refrigerator. If you encounter beauty each time you open your refrigerator door, you will have a natural incentive to keep it clean and to eat the foods that your body needs most.

Warm Lighting

Another factor that can greatly influence the ambiance and functionality of your kitchen is lighting. Often homes have harsh overhead lights that glare on all who enter. Ideally, you'll have a few different types of lighting so that you can alternate them depending on your needs and the time of day. Invest in lighting that you love—lamps can work in a kitchen, as can beam or spot lights that will give you soft, steady light in exactly the place where you need it.

The way that you light your kitchen will have a dramatic effect on how you work and feel in that space. A change in the lighting situation can encourage you to get in there and start cooking. Soft, ample light can increase your efficiency, improve your mood, and transform your kitchen into a place of peace and hospitality.

Chapter 7

Space to Dine

After you've had a chance to bring some order to the kitchen, you might get the urge to beautify your dining room as well. This chapter offers suggestions for making your dining area (whether it be a separate dining room or built into your kitchen) serene and hospitable. This chapter will also suggest an organized, simplified approach to entertaining. And after the guests have left and you're struggling to get the chocolate sauce and wine out of the white tablecloth, you can refer to this chapter for quick cleaning tips.

Determining Your Needs

There are no rules about how to use your dining room. It is your space, and you need to trust your own instincts about how it can best be put to use for your family. Depending on the size and lighting, it could potentially be a great place for homework, meetings, and even a small home office. Even if you don't technically "work" from home, everyone needs a place for sorting through bills and managing paperwork. Your dining room could very well serve this function. Keep in mind, however, that you'll want to be able to conceal stacks of papers and bills so that meals can be peaceful.

As you think about how you can best use your dining space, you might want to keep the following questions in mind:

- What will the primary use of this room be? (Casual dining with your family? Formal dining with friends, family, and/or business associates? Storage? Will this room double as a place for you to do work or your kids to do homework?)
- How often will you use the dining area for dining? (Nightly, weekly, monthly, once a year? Only for holidays?)
- How often will the dining area be used for activities other than dining?
- How many people will you typically need to accommodate? While you may have all of your relatives over each year for Thanksgiving dinner, for example, during the rest of the year, will you typically only have four or six people dining in this room?

After you've assessed your needs for this space, you'll be better prepared to come up with a plan for using it. If you are going to use it for homework or a home office, consider investing in baskets, a filing cabinet, or some other system that can serve as a paper sorter. If your dining room will double as a workspace, keep in mind that it will probably attract massive amounts of paper, so you'll want to be prepared to make quick decisions about how to store (and when to recycle) your paper before it grows from stacks into mounds into mountains.

The All-Important Dining-Room Table

The main piece of furniture in a dining room is, of course, the dining-room table. While it seems as if keeping this room organized would be easy, you are up against one big challenge here. Flat surfaces tend to attract clutter, and this can be especially true with a rarely used dining-room table or sideboard. If you want to make your dining room a place for entertaining and festive family meals, you're probably itching to get that clutter under control.

Be prepared for the reality that you're going to want to stash paperwork, half-finished school projects, and all manner of clutter on that lovely flat surface. This area, which often becomes what the FlyLady would call a hot zone, will need special attention to keep it clutter-free.

If you can keep your dining room in order, however, you'll find that it can be a place of refuge and peace, and that you might feel more excited about the idea of entertaining. You might need to make a commitment to yourself to do a nightly dining-room check, to remove all papers and other clutter on a regular basis before it accumulates. This small, regular effort will pay off when you find you want to use that table!

Another way to keep the paper clutter at bay is to do something that will make your table lovely—put out a bowl of fresh seasonal fruits or a nice tablecloth. When possible, bring in flowers from your garden and arrange them on your table. These items can serve as a reminder that your dining table should stay as clean and beautiful as possible. Beauty and order are closely related. When you seek to make different corners of your home beautiful, you are all the more likely to feel energized about keeping them orderly.

Storing Fine China

Perhaps your dining area has built-in storage or a stand-alone storage piece. This storage can be useful if you are intentional about items you place there. Not only can you keep fine china separate from your everyday dishes, but you can also keep part of this storage empty so that you have a place to stow papers and other items when company is coming.

If your cabinet has glass doors, your china will be pretty well protected as you show off the beauty of your pieces. If your fine china will be stored in drawers or closed cabinets, however, you'll want to take steps to properly protect these expensive and fragile items. Using quilted vinyl cases for china, for example, will help keep dust away, and at the same time will help prevent chipping and scratching.

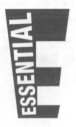

To prevent chips and scratches while storing china in these padded vinyl cases, a separate soft-foam protector is placed in between each item. These cases can then be safely stored in a drawer or cabinet. Dinnerware storage pouches, manufactured from quilted cotton with acrylic felt inserts and zippered tops, can be purchased from Old China Patterns Limited by calling 800-663-4533 or by visiting the company's Web site (*www.chinapatterns.com*).

If a piece of your fine china, crystal, or formal flatware happens to break, chip, or get badly scratched, and your pattern or design has been discontinued, you can find companies that buy and sell discontinued china patterns and other formal dinnerware. Many of them are listed on the Set Your Table: Discontinued Tableware Dealers Directory Web site (*www.setyourtable.com*).

Lighting Options

Just as changing the lighting in your kitchen can transform the space, a fresh light fixture in the dining room can also help make the space more welcoming. A change in lighting doesn't have to cost you much, but it can dramatically transform the way a space feels.

Dual-Purpose Lighting

If you're planning to work and entertain in this space, you might want to invest in at least a few different types of lighting. A floor lamp can be just right for working on your laptop computer, especially if you have a cozy chair in the corner of the dining room to curl up in.

For above the table, there are benefits to a chandelier. Soft lighting is much better in this space than harsh overhead lights. If the light shines up toward the ceiling and then reflects back down on you and your guests, this will be more flattering than a straight-down beam.

As a general rule, you'll probably wind up centering your dining room table directly under your chandelier (or other hanging lighting fixture). In an attempt to redesign the room on a budget, try angling the table diagonally in the room, or pushing one side against the wall (you can pull it out when company comes) to create a different effect.

Typically, when you're hosting a formal or romantic dinner, you'll want mood lighting. You might install a lighting fixture with lights that can be dimmed. You may also want to incorporate decorative candleholders on the dining-room table and walls, if you choose to use candlelight.

The Cost of Lighting

When choosing lighting for your dining area, you have many options. A simple lighting fixture may cost under $50, while a fancy chandelier could cost anywhere from $100 to several thousand dollars. Chandeliers that accommodate 200 to 400 watts provide an abundance of overall illumination. Install the fixture 30" above the table to allow for ample headroom when standing.

The diameter of the fixture should be 12" less than the overall width of the table. Matching wall mounts or recessed lights can also be used to add accent and sparkle. If you purchase a chandelier with a dimmer switch, ask if it might "buzz." This irritating sound can compromise the ambiance created by low lighting.

Easy Enhancements

You can easily enhance the appearance of many formal lighting fixtures by using flame-shaped bulbs in traditionally designed lighting fixtures or using globes or tubular bulbs in contemporary lighting fixtures. Clear bulbs are best with crystal, clear, or other transparent fixtures, and with glass shades. Frosted or coated bulbs work the best with opal, etched, and other translucent-glass shades or diffusers.

If you have artwork to showcase in your dining area, or you want to proudly display your fine china that is enclosed in a display case or positioned on a shelf, you can do so with accent lighting. Think in terms of a few meaningful objects that will create visual appeal. Even if you have many lovely items, too many packed together will detract from the overall effect.

Direct more intense light levels onto artwork or sculptures with directional wall, ceiling, or recessed fixtures. For help in choosing the appropriate lighting for your dining area, visit any lighting specialty store, hardware store, or home-improvement store.

Orderly Entertaining

When planning a formal gathering, it pays to work through the details beforehand. For example, make sure that there's always a clear pathway between your kitchen and the dining area. If you'll be traveling back and forth between these two rooms, choose a seat at the table that's the closest to the kitchen, so you avoid disturbing others each time you leave your seat.

Entertaining can be overwhelming, but you can greatly simplify your task if you ask yourself some questions beforehand. These questions can help guide your decision-making process as you prepare for your guests.

Questions to keep in mind:

- What is the purpose of the gathering?
- Will this be a casual or formal dining experience?
- How many people will be attending?
- What will the complete menu include?
- Do I have enough seating, dishes, flatware, glasses, and serving items to accommodate all of the people attending the event?
- What will the schedule for the event be—when will I serve drinks, hors d'oeuvres, each course of the meal?
- Would a buffet be preferable to a sit-down meal, given the nature of the gathering and the number of people I'm inviting?
- What will the theme of the event be? Do I need special decorations?

As you think about these questions, you'll be able to plan an event that is suited to your needs. Be creative as you plan your event, and enjoy the process. Charles Pierre Monselet, a French author, described the process of preparing a meal this way in a letter he wrote: "Enchant, stay beautiful and graceful, but do this, eat well. Bring the same consideration to the preparation of your food as you devote to your appearance. Let your dinner be a poem, like your dress."

A Simple Affair

Even if you're not Martha Stewart, you can enjoy hosting people in your home, and you can put your guests at ease with the relaxed, hospitable atmosphere you provide. When the idea of entertaining fills you with dread, it's time to lower your expectations for yourself. Your own attitude toward the event will permeate the atmosphere, so you want to be as relaxed as possible. Sometimes the only way to be calm before company arrives is to cut back on ceremony and accept your own limitations. You might, for example, serve a fork-only buffet. If guests can only use one type of silverware, you are less likely to spend hours cooking and use multiple dishes.

Jazzing-Up Takeout

First of all, there is no law against ordering takeout for guests—just use your own plates to make the meal feel more homey. You can also bring some fresh flowers in from the garden and use a nice tablecloth (perhaps with candles?) to make your home feel more welcoming. Think in terms of seasons as well—you can bring the natural world into your home any time of the year. As Victoria Moran writes:

Let your home be seasonal, with its color and sights and scents revolving as the earth does through her primeval passages. Acknowledge spring by bringing in some pussy willows and changing dark linens and wall hangings for pastels. Salute summer with whites and open windows, autumn with russet tones and cider simmering, winter with chairs turned toward the fireplace, the smell of pine, and the coziness of afghans and long novels.

The Potluck Option

If you feel overwhelmed by the idea of hosting a crowd and feeding them a full meal, by all means, take people up on their offers to contribute food to the gathering—or even let them know up front what you'd like them to bring. Some guests might even want to join you in the kitchen to prepare their dishes. Cooking with others can transform a task that feels like a chore into a joy. Potlucks are a bit of an adventure, because you never know exactly what your guests will come up with—this can be part of the fun, too. Just as all of your guests will bring their own presence into your home for the celebration, so too, they'll have a chance to plan and prepare their own piece of the feast. Keep in mind that potlucks can simplify your life in another way—the guests go home with their own large serving bowls to clean.

Choosing and Storing Table Linens

Before your guests come (and after they leave) you'll want to have a plan for your linens. They can add a lovely touch to the table, but storing them can be a little tricky. Here are some tips for making your linens work for you.

Before you purchase table linen, be sure to know the exact measurements of your table. Pay attention to the shape of the table on the package—it can be easy to find the perfect table linen that won't actually fit when you get home. A formal tablecloth should hang down from the edge of the table-top approximately eighteen inches.

Refrain from storing fine table linen in the original plastic packaging it may have been sold in. A plastic container or bag will trap moisture and bacteria, which could eventually cause discoloration. Also, don't store your table linens so tightly folded that they crease. Keeping a tightly folded tablecloth in an overcrowded drawer, for example, will damage the fabric over time.

If you're about to invest in an expensive tablecloth, begin your table-linen collection by choosing a classic white linen or classic damask tablecloth, along with a matching set of napkins. You can later expand this collection with a solid-color cloth that matches an accent color in your dinnerware pattern, for example.

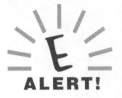

ALERT!

Linens alone will not protect your table. Purchase table pads to go beneath a tablecloth. These pads will greatly extend the life of your table and decrease your own panic when a hot item is set down on the table or a glass of wine spills.

Don't be afraid to wash real-linen tablecloths and napkins in your washing machine. Just set the washer to delicate and use cool water. Fine linen improves in appearance and feel with every wash. Just as you would with expensive bed linen, iron your table linen while it's still damp, on the back side. This will help prevent any shiny patches from forming. Make sure the iron isn't too hot. When storing fine table linens, always launder and iron (or professionally clean) them properly before putting them into storage.

Caring for Flatware

When washing your fine flatware, use only warm, sudsy water. Carefully rinse away traces of food from the flatware. Avoid using harsh dishwashing detergents that contain chlorides. Also, avoid lemon-scented detergents, which contain acids that may harm the metal. It's also important to hand-dry silver, especially knife blades, to avoid spotting and pitting.

If you'll be washing both silver and stainless-steel flatware in the dishwasher, don't put them in the same basket section. You want to avoid allowing one metal to touch the other.

While sterling silver is beautiful, it tarnishes over time. There are many different metal polishes on the market. Some polishes can be corrosive, so take care to follow the manufacturer's instructions.

Keeping your flatware shining is one aspect of the "glory work" involved in making your dining space work. While it can be a headache, it can also be satisfying because the results are almost immediate—polishing your flatware can feel like getting a whole new set for just the cost of the polish.

If You Have a Liquor Cabinet

Whether you have a stand-alone liquor cabinet or a wine rack built into your buffet or credenza, keep all of your related supplies together in one area. In addition to the actual bottles of wine and liquor, some of the supplies you'll want on hand in or near your liquor cabinet include a bottle opener, bottle stoppers, cocktail napkins, cocktail shaker, corkscrew, decanter, foil cutter, ice bucket, pitcher, wine glasses, shot glasses, and a bartender's mixing guide. Some wine racks have special shelves or cabinets to store these accessories.

By paying special attention to how you arrange and keep your dining space, you can create a room that has ambiance, charm, and order. The more care you put into making your dining room lovely, the more joy you will find in the meals you share there with your family and friends. This joy can extend to other areas of your life as well. As Virginia Woolf said, "One cannot think well, love well, sleep well, if one has not dined well."

Chapter 8

The Living Room:
A Space to Gather

The living room tends to be a hub of activity in any home—people gather there to watch television or study, children play there, guests are entertained there. As a result, many living areas become centers of clutter and confusion. This chapter will explore a few methods for making your living space orderly, inviting, and serene.

The Plan for Your Living Room

Because this room is a meeting place where everyone in the house goes, it can often get bogged down with "stuff." Julie Morgenstern reduces the problem to a very basic root—so much goes on in the living room, yet many people do not assign "homes" to the clutter. If, for example, your children play in that room but all of their toys are still relegated to their bedrooms (with the expectation that they—or you—will carry these items to their room every night), it might be wiser to put a toy basket in the living room so that putting toys away will be less of a challenge. If you like to read in this room but the books, newspapers, and magazines tend to pile up on the coffee table, you could think in terms of a few baskets—one for paper products that are ready for the recycling bin and another for those publications that you're still reading.

Before going out and investing in all-new living-room furniture, try rearranging the furniture you have now and accenting or accessorizing to create a whole new look in the room. Simply by rearranging the furniture into a more functional design, and perhaps adding new curtains and lamp-shades, you can create an entirely new room for little or no money.

Perhaps arrange the furniture to face the window or the fireplace (if you have one), or arrange it in clusters to create "conversation centers." This third option could be especially useful if you entertain frequently. Clusters can create a warm and inviting feeling. Also, make good use of alcoves and windows—Julie Morgenstern says that the space surrounding windows is often the most underused space in a home. Could you install bookshelves surrounding the windows, or a low bookcase behind the sofa?

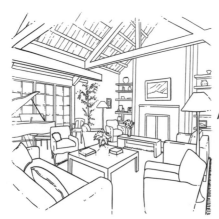

A living room featuring conversation clusters.

Clarify the overall purpose and main functions of your living area, and then consider which living-room furniture pieces you currently own, and which you're interested in adding, based on your needs. For furniture, less is more, so choose pieces that will be best utilized within the room. Could you purchase a coffee table or ottoman that opens up to reveal storage? A sofa that contains a stow-away bed for guests? Especially if you live in a small space, you'll want to think in terms of furniture that can meet a variety of needs.

Organizing Your Entertainment Center

If you'd like to keep your television and related items in an entertainment center, keep in mind that finding the best spot for such a large item is not always easy. When choosing a wall unit or entertainment center, first inventory all of the electronics that you plan to store on and in it. Does this piece of furniture have ample room for your equipment—television, cable box, DVD player, VCR, stereo, video-game system(s), surround-sound system, and speakers (left, right, and middle)? Are there enough electrical outlets located in the area? Will the unit hide all of the wires that go with your electronics? Is there a nearby phone jack? If you'll be using WebTV, TiVo, or certain other types of electronics, you'll need access to a phone jack and probably don't want phone wires running across your living area. Be sure, too, that any furniture that will house electronics is well ventilated, as electronics produce a fair amount of heat.

After your entertainment center/wall unit is in place and you begin to add your various pieces of audio and video electronics, be sure to label all of the wires associated with each piece of equipment. Use a Brother P-Touch label maker (available from any office-supply store) or a pen to write labels on tape that can be wrapped around each wire. You can use different colored ties to wrap related wires together for easy identification.

Living-Area Storage Tips

Storage in the living area can be a tricky thing. First, determine what you need to store, and then be creative. For CDs, DVDs, video games, and video-cassettes, you can purchase a display rack/organizer that holds your entire collection. This can be a freestanding unit, one that is mounted on a wall, or one that fits in your entertainment center or wall unit. If it's a freestanding unit, you might place it in an unused corner of a room so that you can better utilize this space.

You may also want to invest in a multifunctional, universal remote control so that you can replace the separate remotes for your TV, cable box, VCR, etc. with one unit. An alternative is to place a remote-control caddy on the coffee table or near the TV, to help you keep track of your different remote-control units.

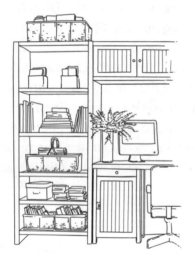

Add baskets to a low shelf for instant storage.

Displaying Artwork and Collectibles

Displaying a collection of artwork, statues, trinkets, memorabilia, or collectibles can be tricky, especially in limited space. Begin by going through your collection and throwing away items that are broken or that you no longer wish to keep. Next, pick out any items that you want to store, but don't want to display at present. You want to avoid making your display look cluttered, because this won't be visually appealing. For the most dramatic visual impact, display just a few items that you really love. Don't be afraid of white space on the walls, either. White space can give the eyes a welcome break from visual clutter and can make a room feel larger.

When hanging pictures or artwork, try to keep them at eye level, and group them fairly closely together. Large gaps between artwork can sometimes be unattractive—instead of creating a feeling of space, the white between images can appear as "dead space."

Make sure your collections or items are properly lit and that the display you create is visually appealing and lacks clutter. According to some interior designers, the secret to elegant displays—even when working with everyday objects—is lush layering. To create your own elegant displays, begin with one tall object that you place in the center of the collection, and then loosely create a triangle shape as you add progressively shorter items to the display. If the items need wall space to be displayed, you might want to fill a blank wall with multiple items with a similar theme (in matching frames, or frames that are similar in style).

Personal Libraries

Some people choose to place personal libraries in the living area. This can be done with relative ease by installing bookcases and/or shelving for this purpose. Your bookcases can be freestanding units, or you can have a bookcase or shelving built directly into a wall. Be sure that the shelving can support the weight of the books. If bookcases seem unstable, you can bolt them to the wall.

To create a well-organized personal library, begin by sorting through your entire collection. Weed out books you no longer want and give them away to friends or donate them to a local library, thrift shop, or hospital.

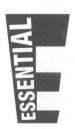

Julie Morgenstern recommends that you take care when arranging your bookshelves. Try grouping books of a similar category together. Likewise, oversized books do not require their own shelves. They can be placed on their side so that more shelves can fit into a smaller space.

Keep in mind that books do not need to fill your entire case. A little empty space in a bookshelf can provide a feeling of spaciousness or create an opportunity for variety—you could place a small sculpture on your bookcase, for example. Also, by leaving some empty space in your bookshelf, you convey to yourself and your family that there is still room to grow—your bookcase can accommodate the needs of a growing family and growing minds.

Fireplaces

Many people love the sight and feel of a fireplace in their living room. While a fireplace can create wonderful ambiance, keep in mind that a certain amount of organization and maintenance is necessary for both wood and gas fireplaces.

Wood fireplaces are beautiful and cozy, but they don't burn as clean or efficiently as natural gas. With wood, you'll need to purchase high-quality fireplace implements—cheap substitutes can bend and burn and be a hazard when you're trying to adjust the position of larger, heavier logs.

Woodpiles are best kept outside, because critters (such as mice and chipmunks) love wood as much as humans do. Ideally, you'll want to bring just a few logs in at a time and place them in a bin beside your fireplace. A covered porch is an ideal spot for storing wood during the winter. If you have no porch, a tarp can help keep your wood dry and ready to burn.

In colder climates, glass doors will dramatically increase the efficiency of your fireplace, because glass doors help to decrease heat loss. Make sure that your damper is in good condition and is kept closed when the fireplace is not in use. If you use your fireplace often, you will want to take care to clear out the ashes under the logs, although if you allow a few layers of ashes to remain, your fire will be warmer and burn better.

In newer homes, gas fireplaces are becoming increasingly common. While gas fireplaces do require much less maintenance than their wood counterparts, you still want to take care to maintain your gas fireplace properly. Be sure to follow the instructions in the owner's manual. Also, take care to have your fireplace inspected annually by a qualified professional service person—gas leaks can be fatal. Although gas fireplaces do not spark, you still want to be careful not to place anything flammable (such as clothing, blankets, or pillows) near your fireplace—the heat could cause a fire. If your fireplace has a glass door and the glass breaks, do not use the unit until the glass has been replaced.

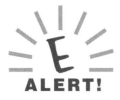

ALERT!

A well-running wood-burning fireplace requires a bit of planning on your part. Use only seasoned wood that has been dried for at least two years. The harder the wood, the better—oak and ash burn well, but pine can leave a dangerous residue in your chimney that can start chimney fires.

Fire Safety

Always use a screen when using a wood-burning fireplace, as hot sparks can be a hazard to your home. Likewise, keep rugs, furniture, and blankets away from your fire, as they can easily ignite. Sparks can sometimes sneak through even the best fireplace screens, so be careful not to let your fire burn unattended. Never leave children unattended near a fire, and keep matches and lighters out of reach (and sight). Also, if you use your fireplace often, you'll want to have a professional chimney sweep come at least every three years to inspect the condition of your chimney. Make sure that the top of your chimney has a screen to keep pests out.

Fireplace Efficiency

Although fireplaces do produce heat, many of them lose as much heat through drafts as they generate. But there are simple things that you can do to increase the efficiency of your fireplace. If you have a wood-burning fireplace with a damper, make sure that the damper is always kept closed when the fireplace is not in use. You can make sure that the seal on your damper is still working well by closing it and putting a tissue in the fireplace. If the tissue blows around, your damper is no longer keeping the drafts out and needs to be replaced or repaired.

Also, when using a (gas or wood) fireplace, turn down the heat in your home and, if possible, close the door to the room with the fireplace so that room will retain the heat. However, be aware that wood fireplaces can create indoor air pollution. You might want to consider keeping a window cracked to improve air quality.

Living Large in Small Spaces

If you live in a studio apartment, college dorm room, or even a small apartment, space is at a premium. You probably have to use every room or area of your home for multiple purposes. This kind of multitasking can make it difficult to keep clutter at bay. That said, American homes are generally much larger than the space actually needed. In other countries, such as Japan, people are able to create well-ordered spaces (and keep them that way) even when they have very little room.

Multiuse Rooms

In a small home, your living area may also double as your home office, guest room, and dining area. Your kitchen may also serve as your laundry area, and your bedroom may need to provide the majority of your storage space (in addition to being a place to sleep).

Every inch of otherwise unused space should be utilized for storage, so be sure to experiment with the various storage and organizational ideas described throughout this book. Utilize underbed storage, or purchase a loft bed so that you can keep drawers and shelves—or create an office area—beneath it.

You may want to build a window seat with storage beneath it, or put cushions on top of a sturdy wooden storage chest so that you can create a comfortable place to sit as well as storage for linens, sweaters, and other bulky items.

Organize your living space into areas or zones by using room dividers, large plants, or bookcases to separate your dining area from your living area or home-office area. A well-built sofa bed can be used as a couch by day and a bed by night to save additional space; just make sure you have a quality mattress.

In smaller living spaces, instead of a full-sized couch and coffee table, you may be able to better utilize your living area by using a love seat or two recliners, plus a set of smaller tables that can be moved around as needed or placed side by side to create a full-size coffee table to accommodate guests. That said, don't be afraid of having a few large pieces of furniture. These pieces can create comfort in a room and provide a focal point for your eyes.

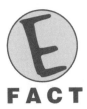

FACT

A small space may not appear larger if you paint it a bold color, but if you love bold colors, don't shy away from them—the trick is to make a space your own no matter what size it is. Bold colors can add dramatic flair and coziness to even the smallest rooms—making them look as if they are "supposed" to be small.

As you design and decorate your living space, focus on your priorities and living habits. Allocate the most space to the activities you do most within your home. If you're a student and spend most of your time studying or reading, a desk with a comfortable chair and ample lighting should be a priority. If you spend a considerable amount of time using your computer, consider investing in a laptop computer as opposed to a full-size desktop computer, and then create a computer-workstation area that's comfortable and functional.

Vertical Shelving

In terms of shelving and storage, think vertical. The most underused space in any room is the two or three feet just below the ceiling. Instead of a three- or four-foot-tall bookcase, think about a seven-foot-tall one. If you can, mount shelves high up on the walls, over windows and doors, and above kitchen cabinets.

When purchasing furniture and other items for your small living space, always think foldup, pull-out, and multipurpose. For example, a dining table can also function as a desk. An armoire can be used for storage, but also serve as a computer workstation. A couch-futon can be used to sleep at night, but during the day can double as a sofa.

As you bring order and comfort to your living room, keep in mind that the best way to keep the space orderly is to make sure that you've integrated logical, easily accessible "homes" for all the items that you'll keep in there. As long as you have an easy spot to store items, the clutter won't accumulate. Careful planning and a little bit of maintenance each day will ensure that this space continues to be inviting and restful.

Chapter 9

Organizing the Bathroom

While the bathroom can easily fall into disarray, there are some steps you can take to get it in order and to make regular maintenance simpler. A bathroom—especially one with a tub or shower—should ideally be a place to slow down and escape the frantic pace of life. This chapter offers tips for making your bathroom more functional, attractive, and appealing—a place where you will want to linger and where your guests will feel welcome.

Appreciating Your Bathroom

Because many people work long hours and rush through their morning and evening rituals, the bathroom can easily become messy. The incredible variety of toiletries available only complicates the problem, as most bathrooms have cupboards full of half-used toothpaste tubes, shampoo bottles, and other personal-grooming products. It can be tempting to buy more of these products than we actually need, because they all promise something different. If you have difficult hair or skin, the temptation only increases, along with those half-full bottles littering the bathroom closet and cabinets.

For most people, it can be a challenge to find time to sort through the clutter and to keep the bathroom sparkling. Your bathroom, however, doesn't need to invite chaos. Nor should you feel like cringing when guests ask to use it. By taking just a few moments each day to order that space, it can be transformed from a place of chaos and clutter into a restful, serene retreat.

Be Attentive to Little Things

You do not need to remodel your bathroom to make it presentable. Instead, focus on being attentive to the little things when you're in there—be honest with yourself about what you want to keep and what you want to let go of, and learn to squeeze short cleaning segments into your regular trips into the bathroom.

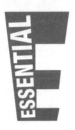

While disposing of half-used bottles of shampoo makes you feel guilty about the waste, keep in mind that products that sit in your cabinet month after month are already being wasted. You might as well forgive yourself for purchasing something that didn't work out and start fresh by getting rid of anything you don't use.

Also, as you begin to tackle the bathroom, think about how you use the space. Although it is possible to modify your habits, try to be realistic about what is actually possible. Sometimes, books on bathroom design will show lovely pictures of glass-fronted cabinets full of neatly folded white towels and perfectly arranged Q-tips, cotton balls, and other toiletries. Although this look might appeal to you, keep in mind the real cost of trying to pull it off. Do you want all your towels exposed? Do you want to spend time folding and smoothing towels so that your display can be perfect, or would you rather organize your bathroom with many simple shortcuts in mind?

This chapter offers simple ways to improve the function and feel of your bathroom. Although this room can be a challenge, it can also be an opportunity. No matter how your bathroom looks at this moment, be encouraged by the thought that with a little bit of regular work and very little cost, it can become quite a different place.

The Comforts of Water

Of all the rooms in your home, the bathroom offers a radically different type of comfort. It offers the cleansing, soothing comfort of water. If your hot-water tank has ever gone out on you, then you've surely realized how we take hot water for granted. As plain and practical as hot water is, it is also one of life's great luxuries.

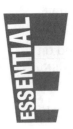

Victoria Moran, on bathing: "Block out time for it on your appointment calendar. Decide what you want from this bath: Do you want to pamper yourself? Prepare for a social gathering? Think through a knotty problem? Soothe aching muscles or stiff joints? Orchestrate your bath accordingly."

Whether your bathroom is tiny and outdated or large and recently remodeled, it offers essentially the same gift to you—a place to shower or bathe, a place to pamper yourself, and a refuge from the rushed pace of life.

Regular Maintenance

On your first bathroom run, you can do something as simple as throw out two empty shampoo bottles. While this may seem like a tiny thing (and the effort is indeed minuscule) you'll find that a little less clutter will make the bathroom feel a little more spacious. On other trips to the bathroom, you can quickly wipe down the yucky tiles around the toilet, clean the mirror, or pick up a few towels from the floor. You don't need to spend two days cleaning your bathroom to make it shine. Think instead of spending a few moments each day attending to specific problems in the bathroom.

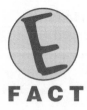

FACT

The FlyLady suggests that you can actually clean the tub ring while you're in the tub: "All it takes is a little bath soap on a washcloth, not cleansers to get it wiped right off. This is when the 'Do it now' principle kicks in. Ten seconds while you're in the tub saves a lot of bending and backache when you're fully dressed."

Although the FlyLady suggests using a little bit of soap to clean the bathtub ring, an alternative that can get your entire bath clean and soothe aching muscles is to keep a box of baking soda beside the tub. If you add a generous amount to your bath—about a quarter box, you'll be able to soothe sore muscles and clean the tub at the same time. While relaxing in the tub, you can scrub down the sides of the tub with the baking soda. Baking soda is an effective cleanser (and can even be used on your teeth), but it is also gentle and nonabrasive. Learn more about simplifying cleaning in Chapter 18.

Because keeping the bathroom orderly can be a huge challenge, try to break the work down into small, manageable steps. Make bathroom maintenance a regular part of your routine and it will become less burdensome for you. Remember what the FlyLady says: "Even imperfect housework blesses my family."

Taming Toiletries

Reorganizing a bathroom can be a pretty major project, so do one bathroom at a time, starting with the most used bathroom in your home. Divide up the bathroom into sections (countertops, cabinets, shelves, shower, closet, and so on).

Begin with the basics: toiletries. Most people have a cumbersome collection of toiletries that they just don't use. Perhaps you purchased an expensive shampoo a year ago that did not work for your hair, but guilt has caused you to hold on to it. If it doesn't work for you, clear it out!

You might have a friend or neighbor who could enjoy the product. Offer it to them. If they turn you down, drop it into the garbage. If you live in a city with alleys, you might place these items in a box beside your dumpster. Somebody might actually come by and choose to take your half-used bottles.

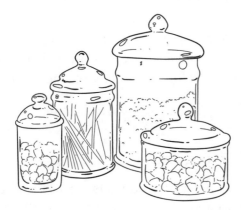

An artful display of toiletries.

There comes a time in the life of every tube of toothpaste when you just can't squeeze any more out of it. You twist and prod and poke, knowing there is at least a few good drops left in there, but they won't come out. Now is not the time for guilt or shame. Just toss those abused tubes into the garbage. Tomorrow morning, you'll be glad to have just one full tube available to you, instead of several mostly used tubes. Your energy is better spent decluttering than agonizing over a few drops of toothpaste.

Although a few old toothbrushes can be kept on hand for cleaning grout and other hard-to-reach places, don't hold on to too many, as they probably won't get used all that frequently. Cleaning with toothbrushes is just a little bit too labor intensive to do it on any kind of a regular basis. Also, make sure that you clearly mark old toothbrushes that you plan to use for cleaning with a permanent marker.

As you shop for toiletries, try to practice no-net-gain. If you buy a new bottle of shampoo, throw out a mostly used old one. If you buy a new tube of toothpaste, get rid of the tubes you're not using. Ideally, every time you place something new in your cabinet, you'll take something out, so that you're not increasing the bathroom bulk each time you shop. Also, the less you keep in your bathroom cabinet, the better. While you'll need room for essentials, a disorganized cabinet can cause you to purchase items that you already have. You want to be able to open the cabinet door and quickly assess both what you have and what you need.

Thoroughly purge just one section at a time. Be aware that you might be tempted to tackle more than you can in the limited time that you have, and resist the temptation to immediately empty every closet and cabinet. If the project becomes too big too fast, it can quickly become overwhelming and unmanageable. As the FlyLady says, "Never take out more than you can put back."

Bath-Linen Organization

After you've had an opportunity to clean out cabinets, closets, and under the sink, think about smart ways to store your towels and washcloths. If they often end up on the floor, this might be because you haven't simplified storage enough. Some towel racks are a hassle—they aren't anchored properly in the wall, so they slip off if any family member grabs them roughly, or they require that you carefully fold the towels to hang them. If you know that you simply don't have the time or inclination to labor over your towel racks, consider a simpler approach.

For example, hooks are a great way to keep your towels. Instead of having to stop and fold your towels, you can simply drop them on the hooks. Hooks require no uniformity and no formality, yet a line of towels hanging on hooks can look reasonably tidy. Just make sure that you install enough hooks so that each family member can fit a towel on a hook without straining the anchors in the wall. Wet towels can be heavy, so you want to be sure to properly attach the hooks to the wall.

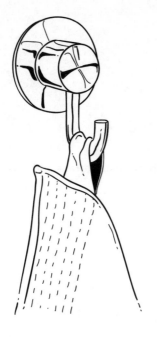

Hooks can help keep your towels orderly without the need to fold and tuck.

Another option with towels is to buy two cubes or bins. In one bin, you can neatly fold towels that haven't yet been used. This cube filled with unused towels can be as lovely as it is practical. The other cube could be used as a hamper for used towels. Especially if your towels are all the same color, this kind of touch can add aesthetic appeal to your bathroom, while increasing function.

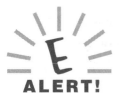
ALERT!

You might need to label some hooks "Fresh towels" and others "Just used." You can also assign a hook to each member of your household. You might even want to designate a "guest" hook. While you may feel comfortable using the same towel for a few days, you don't want to accidentally give a guest a towel that isn't fresh.

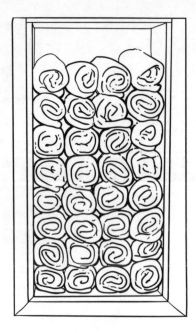

Built-in cubbies create storage and add ambience.

General Bathroom Storage

When organizing your bathroom's cabinets, begin by taking everything out and dividing the contents into defined categories—prescription medications, nonprescription medications, first-aid supplies, hair-care products, makeup, toiletries, and so on. Take mental notes about what kind of organizational accessories may be useful.

The items that you use every day should be placed in a prominent, easily accessible location. If you have a cabinet under the sink, utilize this storage space for items that aren't used daily or that are too large to fit in a medicine cabinet or on the bathroom counter, such as cleaning supplies, extra toiletries, and your hair dryer.

The Medicine Cabinet

If you want to purge but you're not sure where to begin, start with the medicine cabinet. Old prescription and over-the-counter drugs often stay in the medicine cabinet longer than they should because they were a costly investment. But after a certain time period has elapsed, drugs are no longer effective. Check the expiration dates on all medicines and immediately dispose of those that are past their prime.

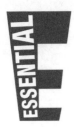

After you've had a chance to bring some order to your bathroom, celebrate by taking a trip to a store that sells organizational tools. Treat yourself to at least one bathroom enhancement—be it small baskets for storing and grouping toiletries or a lovely hamper for your used towels and clothing. These small rewards can help you celebrate your accomplishment.

After you've removed all outdated medicine, study the contents of your medicine cabinet. Purge any items that haven't been used for a year. When the cabinet is empty, clean the shelves and the interior, and then return everything in an easy-to-find order. Separate each family member's prescription medications and place them on separate shelves. Likewise, put all of the over-the-counter medications on a separate shelf. Group all similar items together so that they can be found quickly. There is nothing worse than scrounging for Advil when your head is pounding. Organizing your medicine cabinet is just one more way to care for yourself and your family.

Bulky Items

Your bathroom is not the best storage place for bulky items, such as tissues, toilet paper, diapers, and storage containers filled with extra bathroom items. All of these items can be stored at the bottom of your linen closet. By organizing your space efficiently, you may be able to buy larger quantities of certain items that you use frequently, saving yourself time, money, and trips to the store.

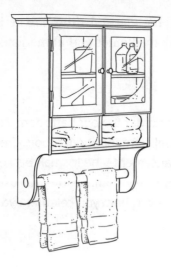

An artful display of toiletries.

Controlling Mold

Mold is a problem in many bathrooms, because the space is often small and not well ventilated. You can reduce mold by keeping a window open, especially when you're showering or bathing. You may also want to install a properly sized ventilation fan. By removing moist air and drying out your bathroom, a ventilation fan helps to prevent mold and mildew. Some new fans can operate continuously and quietly while using less energy.

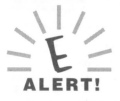

ALERT!

Noxious chemicals in the bathroom may make quick work of tiresome chores, but they can be a real hazard to children, pets, and pregnant women. Even if you have a window in your bathroom, the space is usually so small that you can't avoid inhaling any chemicals that you use.

Old shower curtains can attract streaks of mildew and be difficult to clean. Instead of passively letting the mold grow, however, you can keep an extra shower liner on hand and switch out old shower curtains as soon as they begin to droop and mold. In addition, seal air and water leaks with caulk or expanding foam. You can also purchase a "daily shower spray" to help keep mold and soap scum at bay. These sprays should be used with caution, however. Although they tend to be gentler than heavy-duty shower cleaners, they can still be hazardous to children. You'll want to keep all chemicals out of the reach of small hands.

Lighting Your Bathroom

While few families have money and energy to completely remodel the bathroom, you can drastically improve the mood and feel of your bathroom by adjusting the lights. If you have fluorescent fixtures, you might want to replace the bulbs with fluorescents that have a warmer glow. Ask about these bulbs at any hardware store. If you have the opportunity and inclination, you might also decide to replace those fixtures entirely with lighting that is more soothing.

Lighting Tips

Ideally, your lighting will be shadow- and glare-free. To create a look that you love, think about the time of day when the light most appeals to you. Some people are early birds and love the bright morning sun, while others enjoy the mellow afternoon light. As you consider different lighting options, think about the quality of light that each fixture offers and check it against the quality of sunlight during your favorite time of the day.

You can even out the lighting around a mirror by placing a sconce on either side of it. You can also increase the coziness of your tub or shower by installing a recessed fixture that is designed to withstand moisture. If your bathroom is often chilly, you might want to place a heat lamp over the shower or tub. This relatively cheap enhancement could greatly increase your comfort.

Economical Lighting

The cheapest way to improve your bathroom lighting is to install a dimmer switch. This will allow you to adjust a single fixture to make it better suited to your needs—you may wish to use the lights in full force on a cold winter's morning, but in the evening, when you want to soak in the tub, you might prefer a dim bathroom with candles. Low lighting can make even a very regular bathroom feel more luxurious.

To save money when replacing the lighting in your bathroom, the EPA recommends using residential lighting fixtures with the Energy Star label. These lighting fixtures provide quality, color, and brightness with compact fluorescent-lighting technology. Some people, however, find fluorescent lights to be unflattering, even the warmer varieties. Make sure you test any lighting options before purchasing them. The look of the fixture is as important as the glow of the bulb. You want to be sure that you're fully aware of the effect of both before purchasing a new fixture.

Clever Storage

After you've had a chance to purge and clean, it might be clear that you do need some additional bathroom storage. As you explore storage options, think outside the box. While you could purchase a shelving and cabinetry unit to go over your toilet, you might also be able to use a piece of furniture from another part of the house. Just keep in mind that any items used in your bathroom will need to be moisture resistant. Wood furniture can be used if it is well sealed.

Installing Cubbies

A slightly more complex way to increase your bathroom storage is to install cubbies. This project will likely require the assistance of a professional carpenter, but the cubbies can be both useful and attractive. A cubby can be installed by cutting a hole into your existing wall. Often, there is a good deal of wasted space inside the walls of your bathroom. You can create shallow cubbies by cutting into the walls, or you can create deeper cubbies by cutting into an existing closet or storage space.

If you place neatly folded towels, plants, or other items in your cubbies, they can become attractive and functional additions to your bathroom. Exposed cubbies do run the risk, however, of causing some headaches, as they become just one more space to keep clean and dusted. You might want to install built-in cabinets that have doors so that you don't have to fret over them.

The Beauty of the Basics

Although many items that you use every day—such as cotton balls, Q-tips, and washcloths—do not seem so lovely at first glance, you don't necessarily need to tuck these items away. For a very small amount of money, you can purchase matching glass jars to store them in. If they are displayed in a set of similar jars, they can have a cohesive, attractive look.

Not only will having these items out on a counter or exposed on a shelf be practical and time saving for you, but these little things can look quite lovely when they're displayed properly. Think about old-fashioned general stores, where all of the items were neatly displayed behind glass. When kept tidy and fairly uniform, the items in the jars provided interest for the eye and an overall effect that was appealing. Just keep in mind that only a very few essentials merit this kind of display. Many items are just too unattractive and clunky to fit the bill.

Finishing Touches

If you've followed the steps in this chapter, your bathroom has probably become a lot more functional and a good deal more attractive. Now it's time to think about the "glory work." Add some finishing touches to this space that has already become more appealing.

After you've settled into a routine of basic, regular bathroom maintenance, you might want to add in a few extra steps. For example, by rubbing the tub faucet with a dry, clean towel, you can make the metal shine. This small task only takes a few minutes, but will dramatically increase the beauty of your bathroom.

Likewise, you can bring some of the natural world into your bathroom. You can purchase hanging candleholders and place these on an untiled wall near the tub. You can alternate tea-light candles with fresh flowers from the garden for a simple, refreshing look. Or, you might bring in some fragrant plants that thrive in moist environments.

While the warm, moist atmosphere of many bathrooms can make mold a challenge, this climate can also be an opportunity to try out some tropical plants that would not necessarily thrive in other parts of the house. Many varieties of orchids, for example, can thrive in your bathroom.

As you tackle your bathroom, keep in mind that this project is ongoing and it doesn't have to be labor intensive. A little bit of regular maintenance can keep the larger messes at bay. Encourage yourself to be consistent, but do not demand perfection. Just continue to take little steps each day toward making your bathroom a serene space where you live more fully, linger a little longer, and find the refreshment your soul and body need.

Chapter 10

A Serene Bedroom

Because of the frantic pace of life, bedrooms should be some of the most neglected rooms in the house. In the daily rush, clothes get piled on chairs, pillows are tossed in all directions, and by the end of the week people have to dig a path to find their bed. But this is not the way a bedroom has to be. At the end of a long day, your bedroom can be a place of quiet and refreshment. This chapter will explore ways to make the most of your sleeping space—how to organize your clothing, select and care for linens, and how to create a bedroom that is conducive to rest and nourishing for your soul.

Taking a Clothing Inventory

Most people have a good deal more in their dressers and closets than they actually need. This is especially the case with women, who may have as many as four different sizes of clothing because their bodies shrink and expand. Many women hold on to "skinny clothes" with the dream that they'll one day fit back into them, while also resigning themselves to the reality of those not-so-skinny clothes that also need to be kept, just in case surprise expansions occur.

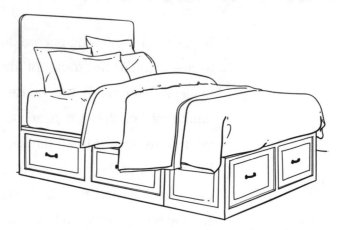

A bed with storage beneath can be both functional and attractive.

Overstuffed drawers and closets, however, create headaches. Finding clothing in the morning can be a huge hassle. The last thing you need when you're struggling against the clock is to have to sift through piles of wrinkly clothing. If you can thin down the contents of your dressers and closets, however, you'll find that getting ready in the morning is a breeze. You may even find that you don't need to go shopping after all. Perhaps all that you need is actually tucked away in your drawers, just waiting to be rediscovered.

While the idea of organizing your clothing may feel overwhelming, you can break the task down into small steps—perhaps you could try to tackle just one drawer a day (or even a week). As the FlyLady says, "Progress, not perfection, is the goal." As long as you're making steady (even if slow) progress, you're going to begin to feel better about your room.

As you sift through your drawers, set out two boxes, one for "Giveaway/Sell" items, and another for "Store" items. Try to be as realistic as possible. If you haven't been able to fit into your size 4 jeans for a good three years, you might want to let them go, trusting that should you shrink again, you'll certainly be able to replace them—and you'll have a great time doing it!

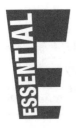

Rule of thumb for clothing: if you haven't worn it for two years, you probably aren't going to start wearing it now. Although it may feel wasteful to toss, give away, or sell an expensive piece of clothing, it is actually a better use of your resources to move that item out into the world where it can help someone else.

Find places other than the closet for storing clothing that you know you'll need but won't be using for several months, such as winter coats, thick sweaters, and other seasonal items. Ideally, you'll move these items to the basement, attic, or storage each time spring rolls around. This small step will simplify your life and help you to feel more at peace in your room.

If you live in a small space without an attic or basement, underbed storage may be an ideal way for you to tuck away off-season items, bedding, or other bulky items. Check stores such as Hold Everything and The Container Store for different storage options. Keep in mind, however, that adding additional storage does come with temptation. You may be inclined to hold on to some items that you'll never use just because you've created space for them. Ideally, underbed storage will be reserved for items that will be useful to you (and that have proven their usefulness over the years).

Bedroom Hot Spots

You may have a few hot spots in your bedroom that could be eliminated. Perhaps there is a chair in the corner, intended for reading, that gets heaped with clothing on a regular basis. Consider moving this chair to a different part of the house so that you (and your loved ones) won't be tempted to drop clothing on it at the end of the day. Heaps of clothing will make you feel discouraged and tired, so it is best to remove furniture upon which clothing can accumulate.

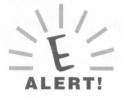

ALERT!

If you want a simple way to keep clothing off the floor and furniture, install a row of hooks in your closet. It takes just seconds a day to "hook" your clothes. With hooks, clothes are easy to spot and putting them away no longer feels like a chore. Take care not to overload your hooks and to only place items on them that will not become stretched as a result.

Removing furniture from your room can have a surprising side benefit. Not only will this make it easier to keep things tidy, but a little less furniture can go a long way toward making a small space feel more comfortable. Keep the primary uses of your bedroom in mind as you evaluate your furniture needs. Rarely used exercise equipment should be shown the door, because in addition to creating clutter, it might make you feel guilty every night as you're drifting off to sleep. Everyone feels burdened enough without the additional trigger of a StairMaster beside the bed. Ideally, the last thoughts of the day will be mellow ones, not thoughts like, "I haven't exercised in weeks. Why did I spend good money on that equipment that I never use?" When you're tired, those kinds of thoughts can be overwhelming, and they might make it harder to fall asleep.

All about Linens

According to the FlyLady, small steps go a long way toward making your bedroom a retreat. She suggests that you invest in a bedspread that you love. With a new bedspread (and possibly linens) you may find fresh inspiration to make the bed every day because you just like to look at it. Also, beauty attracts more beauty. After your bed is made with the lovely spread, you'll naturally feel inspired to keep your clothes off the floor and your bedside tables tidy.

The linens (sheets, pillowcases, comforter cover, pillow shams, bed skirt, and so on) you choose are an investment. If properly cared for, they'll last for many years and provide much-needed comfort as you sleep. To ensure that you experience the most comfort possible, understand what you're buying.

Choosing Linens

When purchasing sheets, the quality and softness are related to thread count. In terms of comfort, the higher thread count you can afford, the better. Although all-cotton sheets breathe well, be aware that they tend to wrinkle more than cotton-polyester blends. Until a few years ago, the best quality sheets had a thread count of 180 threads per square inch. In the past few years, manufacturers have begun offering sheets up to a 700 thread count.

After a thread count goes above 350 threads per square inch, the consumer won't notice a difference in quality. Some foreign manufacturers even use a technique called double-pick insertion to boost thread count, without improving the feel of the cloth. Sheets with a thread count between 250 to 360 threads per inch offer ideal softness.

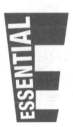

When you wash sheets, take care not to use too much detergent. Over time, too much detergent will harm your sheets. Also, be careful that your detergent is not too harsh and that your dryer is not too hot. These conditions can drastically shorten the lifespan of your linens.

The trick to finding a fitted sheet that will stay on your mattress is to find sheets with elastic that has been sewn all the way around the sheet, not just into the corners. When looking at a sheet's packaging, it should clearly state the mattress size it should fit. There are a variety of non-standard mattress sizes that may appear to be standard but may require special sheets, such as Olympic Queen and California King.

Changing Linens

Before heading to the store to purchase your bedding, determine what your exact needs are for each bed in your home. Ideally, you'll own three sets of sheets for each bed in your home. That way, one can be in use, one in the laundry, and one in storage. Rotate the three sets regularly. Rotating your linens will extend their life dramatically, and by keeping your linens clean, you can eliminate dust mites and other allergens that can make you feel congested and uncomfortable.

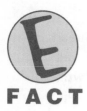

FACT

To save money on sheets, you can buy irregulars. Irregulars often have very small, unnoticeable flaws—or they could have larger problems. You can ask for permission to view the sheets at the store before you purchase them, just to be sure that you can live with the flaws. This is a great way to buy top-quality linens at a fraction of the price.

In addition to having three sets of bed linens and rotating them, another way to make cotton linens last longer is to line dry them as opposed to putting them in the dryer. Also, beware of detergents with too many whiteners—they will compromise the dyes over time.

Storing Linens

When bed linens aren't in use, store them properly. Linens should be laundered before being stored. Sheets and pillowcases, for example, can be kept in plastic bags in a cool and dry closet, out of direct light. To prevent mold and mildew from forming on them, linens should be stored in a way that keeps them away from moisture. Storing the items in a plastic bag also prevents damage from moths or other insects.

Folding linens can be tricky! Here are some steps to follow:

1. Fit one pocket at the top of the fitted sheet into the opposite pocket by inserting your hand behind one pocket and stuffing it inside the other.
2. Smooth the sheet lengthwise and fold lengthwise in half again.

3. Fold the sheets one more time.
4. Store in a plastic bag in a closet, in a dresser drawer, or under your bed in an airtight container.

When storing your comforters and blankets, always launder or dry-clean them first. Also, don't overfold or crush a down comforter or pillow. Allow it to remain as fluffy as possible. Loosely wrap the comforter or blanket in plastic, and then store it in a cool, dry place, such as a closet, a wooden (cedar) storage chest, or an airtight plastic container. To fold thinner blankets, place them in a cotton pillowcase, and then place them in a closet.

Blankets and comforters can also be stored using a freestanding blanket or quilt rack. These are typically made of wood, are placed near the foot of a bed, and provide places to hang various types of blankets out in the open (when they're not actually on a bed). This type of rack can be as lovely as it is functional.

Choosing and Caring for Your Mattress

Many people go for years without replacing their mattresses. This expense can be easy to put off, and the choice of a mattress can be surprisingly complicated. But there does come a time when you notice that you're not sleeping well anymore. You may sleep fitfully at night, or you may wake aching and tired in the morning. Sometimes the culprit is a mattress that is no longer providing the support you need.

It's easy to become overwhelmed when you begin to research beds. In the preliminary stages, ask friends about their beds, about how they sleep at night, and where they purchased their mattresses. You can also read reviews online, although, like the opinions of friends, the reviews are subjective and the reviewers' circumstances (size, physical condition, etc.) may be different than your own.

When you head out to the store, wear loose and comfortable clothing to simulate how the bed will feel when you're wearing pajamas at home. As you test various mattresses, pay attention to the amount of padding and support. Is the mattress comfortable when you're lying down and sitting up in bed? To test a wide variety of products, visit several different mattress retailers and try out at least a handful of different mattresses before making your decision, paying careful attention to the warranty that's offered.

Choose the mattress size you need based on your space limitations in the bedroom and the number of people who will be sleeping on the mattress. For two average-size people, a queen- or king-sized mattress is a must. When determining whether a bed will fit in your bedroom, remember to leave at least fifteen inches on three sides of the bed so you have ample room to move around.

Beds can be expensive, so pay attention to prices. One way to save money is by purchasing a floor model, which is often available for as much as 40 percent off of the retail price. Do be aware, however, that floor models often don't carry the same warranties as brand-new mattresses. Still, floor models are great for people who are seeking a high-quality mattress at a reasonable price. It is often better—in terms of life span of the mattress and comfort—to buy a top-quality floor model than it is to buy a cheaper mattress that has never been used.

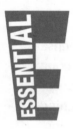

Be a comparison shopper when it comes to mattresses. Depending on the retailer, you may be able to negotiate a better price for your mattress. Ask about floor models and irregulars as well. When you're hunting for a mattress or other furniture, good deals sometimes "hide" and can only be uncovered if you ask questions.

When you buy your mattress, keep in mind that you often get a better deal if you buy both mattress and box spring together. Also, inquire about delivery charges. You might also be able to negotiate these charges. Find out whether there's an additional fee to have your old mattress removed and disposed of. Finally, don't rely on the sales pitch of any single salesperson. Instead, try beds for yourself in the showroom, and then visit other mattress dealers before making a final decision.

Understanding Mattress Options

You have a wide variety of options available when it comes to mattresses. Here are a few options to consider:

Innerspring Mattresses

These mattresses contain springs that are connected in various ways. Whatever the spring design, look for more than 100 coils in a crib mattress, more than 200 in a twin mattress, and more than 300 in a larger model.

The wire gauge of a mattress is also important. In this case, the lower the number, the stronger the wire. Thirteen is the heaviest gauge, while twenty-one is the lightest. You also want to pay attention to the layers of cushioning and insulation that are added to the mattress. The more layers, the more comfortable the mattress will be. If you'd like a cushy surface coupled with firm support below, look for a soft-top model.

Box Springs and Mattress Bases

Innerspring mattresses can be used on many kinds of bases and frames. Typically, the more solid the base is, the longer the mattress will last. A simple sheet of plywood or even the floor can provide adequate mattress support. Besides promoting air circulation, the only advantages of a box spring or other mattress base are the additional resiliency to the mattress and the additional height a second mattress can bring.

Foam Mattresses

A high-quality foam mattress can be just as good as a well-constructed innerspring mattress. The benefit of this type of mattress is that it can be manufactured to fit an odd-size bed. As a general rule, the higher the density of the foam, the better. Ideally you want a minimum density of at least 1.15 pounds per cubic foot in a crib mattress, or two pounds per cubic foot in an adult-size mattress.

Water Beds

Many newer water mattresses come with a solidly comfortable foam edge. Others use an air baffle or rows of springs along the mattress perimeter, and baffles of various designs inside some mattresses slow down wave motion. A polyurethane liner contains the water in case of a leak.

Air Beds

When you think of an air bed, you might think of the squishy pop-up bed used for guests. But there are other types of air beds that can be extremely comfortable. Intex makes a line of Comfort-Rest air beds that can be adjusted to each person's desired level of firmness. These beds are durable, comfortable, and flexible. They also generally have a much longer lifespan than typical mattresses, which last a maximum of ten years. With a high-quality air bed, you could sleep well for as much as twenty years without needing to replace your bed, and you never have to flip the mattress.

Memory Foam

These mattresses tend to be extremely expensive, but some people swear by them. They were developed for use in hospital emergency rooms where burned patients needed the lowest-impact mattress. These mattresses respond to warmth and contour to the shape of your body. While some people love them, others complain that they don't allow for enough mobility during the night, because you tend to sink into one position and stay there for too many hours. Some also say that these kinds of mattresses don't breathe as well as others. But it is certainly wise to try this option, especially if you struggle with back pain; some people have experienced great results through the use of these mattresses.

Protecting Your Investment

A mattress is an investment that should last anywhere from five to ten years, depending on the quality of the product. After the mattress is in place in your bedroom, use a cotton mattress cover as a layer of protection between your sheets and the mattress itself. You'll also want to rotate the mattress 180 degrees at least twice per year, even four times per year or every month. Check with the manufacturer of the mattress for the recommended rotation frequency.

If possible, allow the mattress to air out daily or at least weekly. When you wake up in the morning, remove the blanket and top sheets for at least thirty minutes before making the bed. Also, try to avoid sitting at the same place along the very edge of a mattress too often. Some people sit at the same place on their mattress every morning when getting dressed, for example. This causes sagging to occur faster.

Sleep-Friendly Considerations

Sleep experts are just beginning to understand how the environment in which we sleep affects the quality of our rest. Because we are animals, however, our bodies do respond to primal cues. Too much light in the bedroom can dramatically affect the quality of sleep we experience there. If a street lamp shines directly into your room, you might invest in heavy curtains to block out the light. Did you ever notice how relaxing it is to sleep in a hotel with thick curtains drawn tightly? Hotel administrations have long realized that the quality of sleep their guests experience is critical in gaining repeat or referred business.

Your ability to be productive at work and home—not to mention your overall health—is also related to the quality of sleep you experience. Small enhancements such as high-quality linens and heavy curtains can go a long way toward improving your sleep.

Banish that Desk

Keep in mind, as well, that certain items will interfere with your ability to relax. A desk in your bedroom cluttered with papers, for example, can keep you up and make you uneasy. The worries associated with work and bills don't cease when the sun goes down. The best way to convey to yourself that you're going to let those things go for the night is to push the desk into another corner of the house. That way, daytime duties won't have a chance to bleed into nighttime rest.

Keep It Cool

Also, be aware of the temperature of your room. A room that is too hot will be difficult to sleep in and may even cause bad dreams. A slightly open window, even in the colder months, can go a long way toward moderating your bedroom temperature. A gentle breeze can help increase airflow and help you relax into sleep.

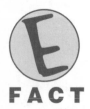

F A C T

Your body moves toward sleep when your temperature drops. This is why a bath before bed (but not immediately before sleep) can be helpful in getting you ready for sleep. Both the bath and exercise will cause your body temperature to rise and stay up for about ninety minutes. After that, your temperature will dip and your body will welcome sleep.

Sleep specialists have also noticed that the things we do in our beds can negatively affect sleep. If, for example, you don't have a desk in your bedroom but you work in bed on your laptop computer during the day, you might find that when you crawl into bed at night, your mind and body will still think "work," not "rest." Ideally, everything in your room will convey a message of rest.

An Intimate Space

Your bedroom is also an intimate space for creating and nurturing life. The best way to make your space conducive to intimacy is to remove clutter. Clear off dressers and bedside tables so that you can enjoy a feeling of space. Odd as this may sound, you might even want to take down personal items, such as photographs and prints. This kind of clutter can make you feel bogged down at night. Try leaving a few blank walls to see if that increases your feeling of rest.

Bedrooms in high-quality bed-and-breakfasts provide a good model for ideal intimate spaces. While they are not overly personalized, they tend to have attractive, comfortable beds, smooth linens, welcoming rugs, and lovely curtains. Elegant touches, such as fresh-cut flowers, enhance the atmosphere. In these uncluttered but cozy rooms, there is space to dream, rest, and love. Everything has a purpose and a place there—and so do you. This is the kind of serenity you can achieve in your own room, one drawer at a time, by becoming intentional about how you organize, dwell in, and decorate your sleeping space.

Chapter 11

Combating Kid Clutter

After you have kids, your life is changed forever. Even before the first little one arrives, gifts from friends and family start to pile up. As the accoutrements accumulate, you can't help but feel overwhelmed, especially if you're striving for a clutter-free home. This chapter explores the task of creating and organizing a kid-friendly room, as well as balancing their possessions and your peace of mind.

Tripping Over Toys

If you find yourself tripping over toys every time you enter your child's room, it may be time to crack down on clutter. Especially in a smaller or shared room, it can be a huge challenge to keep the room orderly if there is just too much stuff in there. Even though your child might be the cause of the mess, you might be surprised by how joyfully many kids react to an orderly environment, especially when you allow them to help develop a system of organization.

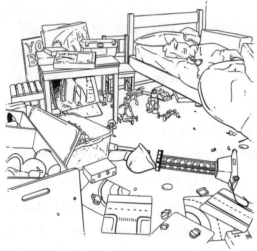

A chaotic bedroom is as disorienting for a child as it is for an adult.

Remember, in your child's room and everywhere else in the house, clutter resists clean and invites conflict. You may find that the sheer volume of clothing, books, and toys in the room creates tension between you and your children. Even if you want to teach them responsibility and make them clean their rooms on their own, they may feel as overwhelmed as you do at the thought of trying to bring order out of the chaos. Children, like adults, probably react to too many items packed in too small a space as if the battle is lost before it has even begun.

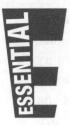

After you and your child have sorted his possessions, reward him by taking him to a store that sells organizational tools and allow him to help you select a few containers. Kids really enjoy putting small items into attractive containers—especially containers that they were able to select. Clear containers will help them to quickly identify what is inside.

Although your child's room can feel overwhelming, the challenge of bringing order to it is also an opportunity. Your child is watching you, trying to determine how to make sense of his environment and how to live well in the space he's been given. Children have little organization practice, and even less knowledge of how to choose what to keep and what to let go of. As an adult who is slowly learning the joy of clutter-free living, you can convey to your child how much better you feel in an uncluttered space, and he might just catch on to the idea.

Post-Holiday Purge

A simple way to start is to not let the holiday season catch you off guard. In between shopping, baking, and preparing for houseguests and travel, take a little time to help your children prepare for the post-holiday onslaught of stuff. If you and your little ones are prepared, you're less likely to be caught off guard.

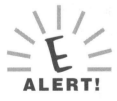

Be sure that the storage in a child's room is easy to use. Drawers that are hard to open will be ignored, as well as shelves that are too high (unless you place a footstool in the closet). Your child's favorite books and toys should be within easy reach, while out-of-season clothes can be stored out of sight.

Try doing either a pre- or post-holiday purge. Let your child know that presents are coming and that he is going to need space for all those gifts. Your child can help make space by letting go of a few items. You might try leaving a box in your child's room marked "Give away" and let him slowly fill that box. Sometimes it is not just the idea of getting rid of things that can be disturbing to a child, but also the quick pace that his parents use for such efforts. By leaving the box in his room, you allow him to take his time and make thoughtful decisions about what stays and what goes.

If you want to sweeten the bait a bit, let your child know that every item he places in the box is likely to be replaced over the course of the holiday season. Especially if your family is large and into gift-giving, it is safe to assume that no matter how many items your child decides to purge, more will come in than go out.

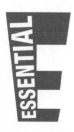

While your child anticipates his holiday gifts, many children around the world have little to look forward to. You may want to encourage your child by explaining how much joy he can bring to others by sifting through his things and picking some high-quality, gently used items to share.

One of the reasons that clutter so easily gets out of control is that we forget to expect it. Certain seasons of life invite clutter. If you're preparing to bring a new baby into the home, for example, you can expect that, although your baby will be small, baby items can easily overwhelm a small space, especially if you haven't taken time to empty-out drawers and shelves before the big event.

Ideally, before a holiday, the birth of a child, the start of the school year, or any event or season that is sure to bring more material items into your home, you can prepare by making space. If you can keep a few empty drawers available, more stuff doesn't have to mean more stress. With a little bit of planning, you can create space for your child's room to grow with his needs.

Planning Your Nursery

If you're about to be a first-time parent, your life will be turned upside down when your new baby is born. Pregnancy is the ideal time to begin to plan a nursery—or to decide if you'll actually need one in those early months. Many parents choose to have their children sleep with them when they're small. These parents feel that they are better able to respond to middle-of-the-night cries when baby is close at hand.

Bringing Down the Bar

If you want to design a separate nursery for your baby, keep in mind that babies don't need or expect much. You do not need top-of-the-line items, but you do want to be aware of safety issues. Old cribs are sometimes unsafe, for example. As you plan your purchases of furniture and fixtures for your nursery, make sure you choose items that meet the safety guidelines issued by the U.S. Consumer Product Safety Commission (*www.cpsc.gov/cpscpub/pubs/chld_sfy.html*).

What You Might Need for a Nursery

A baby's sleep needs will change with each phase of life. When the baby is small, she might sleep in a bassinet or with her parents. When she begins to sit up and roll, a crib might become necessary.

- **Changing table:** Until your child is toilet trained, you're going to be changing a lot of diapers. The area where you'll be changing diapers should be a safe area for your child, plus have storage (shelves or drawers) for all of the items you'll need. While the baby is being changed, everything you need (wipes, creams, diapers, and so on) should be within arm's reach for you, but not for your baby. You don't ever want to turn your back on the child. The changing table should have a concave shape in which you can nestle your child to discourage her from rolling over.

- **Diaper bin:** If you choose to use disposable diapers, you might want to invest ina diaper disposal system, a container that seals each diaper in film, locking in germs and odors. It can be operated with one hand, so you can use it while changing your baby.
- **Clothing hamper:** Many companies offer hampers designed to fit the décor of a child's nursery or bedroom. Baskets, for example, come in different shapes and sizes. Consider purchasing a hamper that will be easy for your child to maneuver (and fun for them to use!) so that they will want to put their own laundry in the hamper.
- **Toy bin:** After your child is born, she will probably start to amass a large toy collection. You'll want to keep these toys organized and tucked away. A toy bin is an ideal way to do this. Pay attention to the construction of the unit and make sure it's totally safe. The lid should not be able to slam shut, nor should it be able to entrap your child.
- **Nursing chair:** A comfortable rocking chair is ideal for nursing an infant. Glider rockers, which gently move forward and back, are soothing for both mother and child. These chairs are also great for reading to or comforting an older child.
- **Smoke detector:** Make sure you install a quality smoke detector in the nursery. Check the battery monthly.

Arranging the Furniture

After the room is selected, think about what your daily routine with the infant will be, and then position the furniture accordingly. Near the rocking chair, for example, you may want a bookcase and a table (where you can place whatever you'll need to nurse the baby). You'll probably also want a telephone with a speakerphone in this area, and you may want to have a view out a nearby window. Keep a dresser containing your child's clothes close to the changing table, so that you can easily reach various garments while dressing your baby. If the clothes will be kept in a closet, you might want to place the changing table as close to the closet as possible.

As you arrange furniture, try to maximize floor space as much as possible. To generate more floor space, utilize lighting that attaches to the ceiling or walls (as opposed to floor lamps) and take advantage of vertical storage spaces (tall bookcases or dressers with drawers stacked vertically).

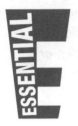

Prior to having furniture delivered, consider how you need to prepare the room itself. For example, does the room need to be painted or wallpapered? What about flooring, window treatments, or electrical work (outlets and lighting)? Before the furniture is delivered and set up, make sure the room is totally prepared and well cleaned. You'll also want to remove all of the clothing, toys, and other items from the room.

Safety Considerations

Always think in terms of safety when planning and organizing your nursery. Be conscious of electrical cords, curtain cords, and toys with small parts or pieces. Never hang artwork, mirrors, or items directly over the crib, where they could fall on your child.

To make certain your nursery and your entire home are properly childproofed, you can hire a professional baby-safety expert who will visit your home and help you organize it. The International Association of Child Safety (888-677-IACS) can offer referrals.

Keeping Up with Clothes

Children's clothing can be a major source of clutter and confusion, especially when children are small and growing fast. While adults merely have seasonal clothing changes, babies and children outgrow clothing and shoes in a matter of months. Add to this the fact that most parents of young children already feel overextended, and you have all the factors that can lead to an organizational disaster.

You might want to go through your child's clothing every few months to pull items that no longer fit. If you're planning to have more children, you can store the outgrown clothing in a box marked with the original owner's name and age or size. If you already have younger children, you can pass along the appropriate outgrown items to whomever they will fit.

Just as you need to be realistic as you sift through your own clothing, try to be as realistic as possible about your children's clothing. There are certain items that may have been gifts or expensive purchases that just did not work out. Perhaps the fabric was too scratchy or the buttons too tricky, or the clothing just never fit right. These items can be given away or stored for future siblings.

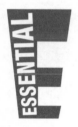

If you chose to store your child's outgrown clothes for future siblings, take care about how you arrange the boxes. Ideally, all boxes will be clearly marked and they'll be lined up by size so that as your next child grows, you'll have easy access to the next-size clothing.

The best way to avoid kid clutter, however, is to be discerning about what comes into your home in the first place. Take care to purchase items that you are certain your child will enjoy wearing. If you have a child with strong opinions, you might be wise to bring them to the store with you and let them weigh in before committing to purchases.

Resorting to Sneakiness

The only way to keep clutter at bay is to keep it moving, especially when you realize how quickly it accumulates. If, despite your best efforts, your child is still a bit of a hoarder and you cannot compel her to place items in the give-away box, you may need to try one of two approaches.

One approach, advocated by the book *Parenting with Love and Logic* by Foster Kline and Jim Fay, is to teach your child to become responsible for her own items. This approach requires a bit of "tough love." Instead of yelling and complaining about messes in your child's room, you can tell her that if she doesn't keep toys and clothes off the floor, those items might just disappear one day.

Especially when your child is small, you'll want to help her work out organizational systems that are logical for her. It is reasonable for her to ask for and expect your help. But as she matures, challenge her to take ownership of her own room.

This approach has two great benefits: it teaches the child to be responsible for her own items—a lesson that lasts a lifetime—and it allows the parents to delegate. A parent who can share the work of home organizing with his child is less likely to feel overwhelmed. A child who feels that she has a share in the household is also likely to feel a boost in her self-image. If you take opportunities to help your child cultivate these kinds of skills, she will be better able to manage her home as an adult.

Another—more sneaky—approach is to use those hours when your child is away at school to declutter the room yourself. This is especially recommended for younger children, who are less likely to be upset by a feeling of having their personal boundaries crossed. When children are older, you'll want to work with them to help them purge. As they age, any "invasion" into their rooms when they're not there will be taken as a betrayal.

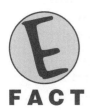

FACT

Although it could be devastating for your child to find that some of her toys have disappeared, it will be more draining for you, over the long haul, to always have to pick up after her. If you follow through with the threat, you'll be surprised at how much more consistent your child will become in her cleaning habits.

Especially when children are small, you may be able to cart-off toys, clothing, and the like without them noticing. You may fear that they'll come home and be devastated by the results of your purge, but instead find that they (like you) are just happy to be in a place that is less cluttered.

Often, after you carry off a few bags of their items, children discover toys that they had forgotten. Many young children will spend hours quietly "rediscovering" their more precious toys that may have been obscured by the clutter. It can be a great joy, for both parents and children, to finally be able to appreciate what they have instead of always thinking in terms of more. Clutter invites more clutter. Things don't look (or feel) right, so you're tempted to try to buy additional things to fix the problem. In an orderly and serene environment, however, contentment will come naturally.

If you're living in a tight space, consider the following space-saving options:

- Add hooks on the closet door(s) and inside the closet (on the side walls) for jackets, shoe bags, and other items.
- Free up valuable floor space by utilizing a loft bed for your child. The sleeping area is on the top, while a desk, dresser, shelves, or other forms of storage space can be built beneath the bed.
- If you need to accommodate more than one child in a room, get bunk beds.
- Install shelving on the walls, as opposed to using a freestanding shelf unit that takes up floor space. On these shelves, store books, toys, collectibles, trophies, and other items.
- Install underbed drawers and use underbed storage bins for off-season clothing, toys, sports equipment, and so on. It may make sense to raise the bed slightly to create additional underbed storage.
- Keep furniture to a minimum. Whenever possible, choose pieces of furniture designed for multiple uses. For example, some children's beds already have shelving or drawers built in.
- Make full use of closet organization tools to best utilize closet space.
- Take advantage of the storage space that a good-sized toy chest provides. This can be a central location where toys are kept. Within the toy chest, use plastic bins or shoe boxes to separate toys with lots of small pieces, such as building blocks, toy cars, board games, action figures, dolls (and accessories), and trading cards.
- Display shelving can sometimes be installed about a foot down from the ceiling line. You can use this shelf space to show off collections, trophies, artwork, and other items that don't need to be readily accessed.

Although basic organization can go a long way toward helping your child live more fully in her space, you can also choose items carefully to best serve the space your child inhabits. Finding the furniture that's well built, functional, visually appealing, durable, and within your budget requires searching. Be prepared to visit a number of furniture stores to see the available options. If this furniture will be used by young children, pay careful attention to the quality of construction and think in terms of product safety.

If you're budget-conscious, shop around by visiting your local furniture retailers (including children's-furniture specialty stores and department stores), and then use the Internet to compare prices from online retailers. It's not a good idea, however, to purchase children's furniture you haven't seen, touched, and examined firsthand.

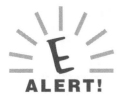

ALERT!

Don't try to save money by purchasing poor-quality furniture or secondhand furniture (especially for an infant or toddler) that may not meet the latest safety guidelines issued by the U.S. Consumer Product Safety Commission (*www.cpsc.gov/cpscpub/pubs/chld_sfy.html*).

No matter where you buy furniture, keep the following tips in mind:

- Figure out your budget and time frame.
- Decide on a basic look, style, or theme.
- As you see what's available, compare value, workmanship, durability, and safety features.
- Keep storage capabilities foremost in mind.

You can utilize several different types of storage in a bedroom, including open storage (shelves and baskets), closed storage (armoires, bins, chests, underbed storage, and dressers), convenient storage (closets), and remote storage (closets and storage options in other areas of your home, such as the basement, attic, or garage).

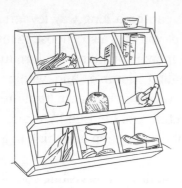

Baskets, cubbies, and cabinets
can increase storage.

Make sure the individual pieces of furniture you choose will fit properly into the layout (both size and décor) of the room as well as into your budget. For example, if you're purchasing a large dresser, is there ample room to open the dresser drawers? After you know the exact measurements of the bedroom as well as the individual pieces of furniture you're interested in, sketch out on paper the room's proposed layout.

Working with a Budget

Based on where you're shopping, furniture prices may be negotiable. Check into floor models and future sales. Determine what extra costs may be involved. For example, does the furniture store charge extra for certain colors or finishes? What are the setup and delivery charges? Does the price you're being quoted include all of the accessories you see in the showroom? Watch out for hidden costs and make sure you understand exactly what you're paying for and what you'll receive.

Based on the costs and your budget, consider purchasing only a few pieces of furniture at a time, putting off buying furniture that you don't need right away. For example, if you're creating a nursery for your newborn baby, you won't need a crib for several months. You can put off this purchase until it's actually needed and use a bassinet in the meantime for the newborn. Some parents also choose to sleep with their babies, an option that can be safe and comforting to the infant, assuming that the parents do not consume excessive alcoholic beverages, are not obese, and do not sleep on extremely soft beds with numerous bulky blankets.

Creating a Nest

Especially when your child is small, he will sleep better in a room that feels like a nest. He does not need the most expensive, elegant furniture. What he does need is to be able to sleep peacefully in a space that feels snug and secure. If possible, move the bed to a corner or alcove where your child can feel "tucked in."

If there are no corners or alcoves for your child's bed, you might want to get a bunk bed. Not only does a bunk bed provide sleeping space for two, but it can feel cozy to a child to be on either the top or bottom. A bunk bed allows for two separate "zones." To your child, it can almost feel like two small rooms within the room. To make the bottom bunk extra serene, try hanging drapes or even sheets from the side of the top bunk. This will create a feeling of security for your child, and will make his sleeping space a little darker, which can hasten sleep.

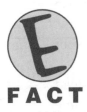

FACT

In *Sleepless in America*, Mary Sheedy Kurchinka says that children generally sleep better when their beds do not "float" in the middle of the room. If you have the space in your home, try to keep sleeping and playing areas separate. If your child's bedroom is full of toys, he may feel tempted to play the night away rather than sleep. When space is at a premium, plan to tuck toys into bins or closets as part of your nightly ritual.

According to Kurchinka, it is wise to limit children's media exposure, especially in the bedroom. The light from a computer screen or television set can be very stimulating to a young child. The activity of watching television, while it may seem to evoke a sort of trance for your young child, can actually keep him awake for hours afterward, especially if the program he saw was too fast-paced or disturbing. The mere presence of a television or computer in your child's room can cause him to stay up later than you want him to.

Be aware of heat, noise, and light. Like you, your child needs to have his body temperature drop for him to fall asleep. He will sleep better in a relatively cool room, bundled under blankets that can be removed if he becomes too hot. Natural fibers, such as cotton, will also allow the blankets to breathe better—your child will stay warm at night without getting overheated and sweaty.

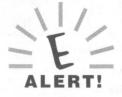

ALERT!

Be aware of potential allergens that may disrupt your child's sleep. Pet dander is often a culprit. Cigarette smoke also is known to cause sleep disturbances for children because it makes it harder for them to breathe. Likewise, down comforters or pillows might exacerbate allergies. Wash sheets weekly in hot water to keep dust mites away.

Depending on the orientation of his bedroom, your child might need heavy curtains to block out the light. These curtains also help in the summer when the long, bright hours can keep your child awake. Some kids are also extremely sensitive to noise and can benefit from a white-noise machine. These inexpensive devices block out the sounds that interfere with your child's ability to sleep.

Streamline your child's room so that its purpose becomes clear—instead of the bedroom being a work or play space, it should be a sleepy space, free from the glaring lights, troubles, and noise of the world. A soothing, uncluttered environment will make your child feel safe enough to rest.

Chapter 12

A Space for Guests

If you frequently host guests, then you know how chaotic it can feel when you're preparing for them. This chapter will explore ways to make your guests feel more comfortable in your home, as well as ways to put you at ease before (and during) their visit. If you take a well-organized approach to hosting guests, you'll be able to relax and enjoy their company—and they'll be able to relax and enjoy a peaceful retreat in your home.

Planning Ahead

If you've been slowly working through the steps in this book, then you're probably beginning to feel a little bit better about the idea of hosting guests. Sometimes people put off guests simply because they feel that their homes are not clean or attractive enough. You have no need for shame, though! Whatever you have been able to accomplish while slowly working through the steps in this book has most likely improved the look and feel of your home.

Keep in mind, as well, that few of guests expect perfection (if you fear they will, you can suggest that they stay at a bed-and-breakfast). Because you live in your home with your family and pets, your home is going to show signs of life no matter how hard you work to keep it orderly. This is okay— your guests have come, at least in part, because they want to experience a bit of your life, imperfections and all. After all, they have the same challenges in their own homes.

Prioritizing

In Victoria Moran's book *Shelter for the Spirit*, she offers this tip for simplifying your life: "Put things with feelings first." Sometimes when you prepare for guests you can let yourself get so stressed about cleaning and cooking that you forget the people who presently surround you. But the attitude that you have about hosting guests will be conveyed to those who know you best. If you're short-tempered and tense, you will convey to your family that you don't really enjoy guests. If you can be calm and prepare for your guests a little bit each day, you're more likely to enjoy your guests and your children will be more likely to behave well when the guests are there.

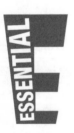

Victoria Moran, on prioritizing: "Balancing your checkbook is probably not as important as listening to your child. Having a romp with the dog should usually take precedence over waxing the kitchen floor. That's because bank accounts and linoleum can wait until a more convenient time. Things with feelings cannot."

The frantic pace of life can make it difficult to plan ahead, but you'll never regret having taken small steps to prepare for guests. As much as you want to graciously host them, be realistic up-front about what is possible. If you live in a major city and have small children and an airport run seems next to impossible, let your guests know a few weeks in advance that they'll need to take a shuttle or taxi to your home. If you provide them with very specific instructions, they should have no problem doing this. It is far worse for guests to sense that they are a burden to you than it is for them to have to exercise some independence.

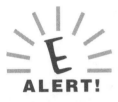

When you plan meals for your guests, keep in mind any dietary restrictions they might have. If they have very specific food needs or preferences, you can take them to the grocery store when they arrive and allow them to be part of meal planning.

If you enjoy cooking and are confident that your guests can eat whatever you serve up, think in terms of make-ahead dishes that you can prepare early in the week and then warm for your guests. Homemade soup with good bread is an ideal choice for that first night, as you often won't know if your guests have eaten during the journey. Soup is light but satisfying, and if your guests have eaten, soup can wait until tomorrow.

Another great dish for guests that freezes well is lasagna. You can make this early in the week, freeze it, and then reheat it when your guests arrive. The best part of make-ahead meals is that you won't need to frantically clean (while cooking) just before your guests arrive. That challenge, especially when coupled with an airport run, is enough to make anyone tense!

Serve Local Fare

If you live in an area that is known for some particular food, try to serve that to your guest. If you live in New York, for example, and your guest enjoys fish, bring in fresh lox and bagels in the morning. If you live in Chicago, plan to take your guest out to enjoy Chicago-style pizza or an eatery in one of the many ethnic neighborhoods. If you live in Oregon, by all means, serve fresh

Pacific salmon—any guest from the East Coast will immediately realize that Pacific salmon offers a completely different culinary experience from its Atlantic counterpart.

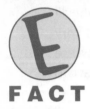

FACT

Eating can be an adventure, especially for your houseguests. "'When you wake up in the morning, Pooh,' said Piglet . . . , 'what's the first thing you say to yourself?' 'What's for breakfast?' said Pooh. 'What do *you* say, Piglet?' 'I say, 'I wonder what's going to happen exciting *today*?' said Piglet. Pooh nodded thoughtfully. 'It's the same thing,' he said."

—A.A. Milne

A great way to show your guests local fare is to take them to a farmers' market that requires that all the farmers be local (keep in mind that many markets allow food that has been shipped in from faraway states). Local markets not only allow you the opportunity to connect with the people who plant and harvest the bounty on your table, but will let your guests see what types of produce, cheeses, and breads are produced right in your own backyard.

After you've thought out some meal possibilities, think in terms of snacks to keep around the house. Crackers, fresh veggies, cheese, fruit, and dip can be nice to munch with your guests while you catch up with them. Guests also sometimes wake hungry in the middle of the night—ideally, they will know which cupboard to dig into for a quick, satisfying snack. If you have the opportunity to bake something fresh before your guests arrive, all the better.

On that first evening with your guests, make sure that they know how the coffeemaker works and where the tea is stored. Show them where you keep cereal and fresh fruit. Some guests (especially those who have traversed time zones to get to you) will wake before you do. You don't need to rush out of bed to help them—just let them know where everything is the night before. They might even appreciate having a chance to wake slowly by themselves while you sleep.

Convertible Spaces

In most people's homes, space is tight. Many people are forced to host guests in the living room. If this is your situation, there are a few things that you can do to make your guests more comfortable. First, if you do purchase a sofa bed, don't go by aesthetics alone! Make sure that you have an opportunity to test the mattress before the purchase is final. If you've found a sofa that you love and is within your budget but you're not satisfied with the mattress, you can buy an extra mattress pad to increase the comfort. You can purchase a Tempur-Pedic mattress pad, or any foam pad at a discount or department store. These small touches can greatly increase your guests' ability to sleep in your home.

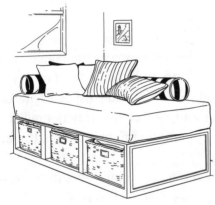

A daybed can provide extra seating, storage, and space for guests.

If you've designated a room to be your guest room, but you don't have guests too often, you probably want to utilize this space for other activities as well. Perhaps you'll use your guest room as a home office, an exercise room, a room to participate in your hobby, a room to display your knickknacks or collections, or a playroom. If the room does have multiple uses, it can be challenging to covert it into a guest space—the mere clutter most of these uses create can make the space feel cramped and unwelcoming.

Ideally, you'll decrease the clutter in that room especially. This will take vigilance on your part because you probably won't have to see the clutter all the time.

One of the greatest temptations with an "extra" room is that this room can easily become a catch-all for the items from the rest of your house that haven't yet found a home. If you plan to use this space for guests, however, you'll want to try your best to stay on top of the clutter. Otherwise, the prospect of guests will feel overwhelming.

If you'll also use this space as a home office or hobby area, think in terms of furniture that can conceal—for example, a desk/armoire that can be closed at the end of the working day is a great way to keep your working space private and to help you set boundaries on your time. When the desk is closed, work for the day has ended and you can relax with your family, just as those who travel to a different physical space are able to at the end of the day.

Create a Peaceful Retreat

Wherever your guests slumber, you'll want to make the space conducive to sleep. Even a living room can be a peaceful place to sleep if you keep a few things in mind. First, can you make your guest space dark enough? Many people sleep better in a dark room, especially in an unfamiliar setting. If you don't own any yet, consider purchasing thick curtains to block out streetlight.

Light that may not be bothersome to you could feel invasive to your guests, so be sure to seek creative ways to solve this problem. If thick curtains are outside of your current budget (or you simply don't like the look of them) you might purchase facemasks (to block out the light) and several pairs of earplugs for your guests. Especially if you have small children, your guests will thank you for those earplugs!

Just as some guests will want complete darkness, others will need a little bit of light. Offer a nightlight and alarm clock to your guest in case these items will be useful. Ideally, the room where the guests sleep will have a variety of light sources so that they can use lamplight to read by at night and brighter lights to dress by. Carefully selected lighting can help create a warm ambiance in almost any room.

The Pet Problem

If possible, keep your pets contained during the nights when you have a guest in your home. Pets wandering the house can be startling for a guest, especially if you have an overly friendly dog or cat that decides to curl up with your guest. Check with your guests to see how they feel about pets before they arrive and plan accordingly.

If your guest has a pet allergy, try to keep your pets away from her sleeping area. It is a good idea to vacuum up pet hair as much as possible, although take care to do this a few days in advance, as vacuuming can stir up dander and actually make it harder for allergic guests to breathe. At the very least, make sure that you have an allergy medication on hand should your guest need a little relief.

Comforting Touches

There are small things you can do that will make a big difference to your guest. In terms of bedding, try to provide your guests with the softest sheets you can afford. The higher the thread count, generally, the silkier the sheets will feel. Flannel sheets in winter are also a nice touch for guests.

Make sure to provide ample blankets for your guests so that they can layer and remove blankets as they see fit. It is best to provide at least two pillows per guest, especially because some people are very sensitive to the flatness or puffiness of particular pillows and it may take your guest some time to determine which pillow she can actually sleep on. Again, check with guests about allergies. Some people love the feel of down pillows, for example, while others will sniffle all night long if forced to sleep on a down pillow—if possible, purchase some allergen-free pillows for guests.

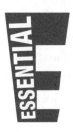

A vase of fresh-cut flowers near your guests' sleeping area can add a welcoming, elegant touch. Likewise, you can leave a stack of books that you feel they might enjoy on a table near the area where they'll sleep. Many people have trouble sleeping in a new space and will welcome the diversion.

Leave fresh towels (two for bathing and at least one washcloth) at the foot of your guest bed. This way, your guest will know that she has fresh and clean towels. If you purchase guest towels in a color other than the one your family usually uses, you will be better able to distinguish which towels are for guest use only.

Room for Guests

Even if you can't provide a separate sleeping space for guests, can you provide a few empty drawers or baskets under a coffee table or some closet space for them? Here is where all of your hard work begins to pay off. Instead of needing to clear out drawers and closet space for guests, you'll likely have some empty spaces just waiting to be filled. A little bit of space to unpack and settle in will allow your guests to feel more at home and will allow them to keep their clothes looking fresh and unwrinkled.

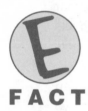

FACT

If closet space is tight, purchase a freestanding clothing rack from any hardware store or mass-market retailer. It's also nice if you can offer your guests a television and/or radio in the guest room.

Furnishing Your Guest Room

If you are in a position to purchase additional furnishings for the guest room, think carefully about what you'll be using this room for in addition to housing guests. Measure the room carefully, and then determine what type of furniture is required to make the room functional. As with all of the rooms in your home, take advantage of organizational products, such as specialty hangers, underbed storage bins, dresser drawers, and shelving to organize and properly store your belongings. To save space in your guest room, you may not want to use a full-size, traditional bed. Keep in mind, however, that there are many space-saving alternatives, discussed in the following sections.

Air Mattress

The AeroBed (*www.thinkaero.com*) is an excellent choice. AeroBed is a self-inflating bed that fully inflates in less than a minute and deflates in fifteen seconds. It has a built-in electric pump for fast, easy inflation. When not in use, it deflates to the size of a sleeping bag and can be stored in a closet.

Futon

The biggest benefit of futons is that they're much more affordable than sofa beds. They're also generally far more sleep-friendly than traditional sofa beds, although they tend to not be as comfortable (or attractive) as sofas. Keep in mind that when unfolded, futons can take up the same amount of space as a full-sized couch or sofa bed.

Sofa Bed or Chair

When not used as a bed, these pieces of furniture double as full-sized couches or oversized armchairs that come in a wide range of styles. When a bed is needed, they typically unfold into a single-, king- or queen-sized bed. Some sofa beds have custom-size mattresses. The cost of sofa beds varies greatly, based on the quality of the couch as well as the type and quality of the mattress built into it.

Keep in mind that some sofa beds can be uncomfortable to sit and sleep on. They also tend to be heavy and extremely difficult to move. Should you choose to purchase a sofa bed, make sure you've inquired about the comfort of the mattress beneath the cushions. If you already own a sofa bed with an uncomfortable mattress, consider purchasing a generic memory-foam mattress topper. This small addition could greatly improve your guests' sleep.

Portable Cot

These metal frames on wheels fold in half for easy storage in a basement and utilize a thin (often foam) mattress. They come in several different sizes and tend to be very inexpensive. Cots are a good option for children, but adults are likely to wake with a sore back after sleeping on them.

Wall Bed

If you're building a home office and want it to double as a comfortable guest room, Techline (*www.techlineusa.com*) offers a home-office furniture system that includes a pull-down wall bed. This system allows you to utilize the room space available to include a full-sized desk, shelves, cabinets, plus the pull-down bed that sets up in minutes. See Chapter 5 for additional information about setting up a home office.

Displaying and Organizing Photographs

Whether your guests sleep in the living room, a guest room, or your home office or hobby room, it is likely that your photographs will be stored somewhere near them. Perhaps they fill a guest-room closet or take up precious drawer space in your living room. In order to create a more orderly environment for your guests and yourself, you'll want to take some time to get your photographs in order.

You can display, organize, and store your personal photographs and memorabilia in many ways. Because you probably don't have enough wall space to frame and hang all of your pictures, consider a few alternatives, such as creating a scrapbook or using labeled boxes for storage.

Organizing Photos and Negatives

Begin by finding a method for organizing all of your photographs, including labeling the negatives, writing about the pictures, and storing the photographs until you are ready to mount them in your scrapbook. After you establish a method, every time you have a new roll of film developed, implement your organizational strategy immediately. You may make a rule to develop your photos within a week of taking them, for example, or to organize the photos in an album or photo box within a month of having them developed.

Also, there are a variety of things that you can purge out of your photo boxes without even having to deliberate. You don't need those floppy envelopes that photos come in, especially if you're going to use a shoebox or albums. Dump these excess items immediately and you'll be better able to sort through the photographs.

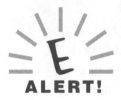

ALERT!

Although it can be tempting to hold on to all of your photographs, extra photos just generate clutter. If you have duplicates of photos you love, send them to receptive friends and family. They'll enjoy the fact that you thought of them, and you'll have a few less objects to keep in order. Also, purge all photos that are blurry or unflattering to the subjects portrayed—your friends and family will thank you for this!

Make sure to keep your photos in a temperature-controlled environment. Basements and attics are unsafe places for photographs. Also, the way that you store your photographs will have a dramatic effect on their longevity. When possible, keep them in plastic bins. Use acid-free labels to date and describe photos. If you're able to store your photographs in a climate-controlled environment, consider professional home organizer Julie Morgenstern's method of using labeled shoeboxes. Shoeboxes don't cost anything and are the ideal size for photographs. You can arrange your photos in a variety of ways—by year, by topic, by vacation—or you can have bins for each member of your family (or each branch of your extended family). Even if you never get around to placing your photos in albums, a basic shoebox system can serve to make them accessible for years to come.

Organizing your photographs can be daunting, so don't try to tackle them all in an afternoon or over a weekend. Instead, make a weekly commitment to a manageable goal, such as creating one shoebox a week. You can even pencil your photo-organizing time into your calendar.

You might also want to create a simple box for pictures and keepsakes pertaining to each family member. These boxes will probably need to be larger than a shoebox if you want to save children's art, report cards, and other larger items. Be selective as you create your memento box. Choose only the best to keep—those that most clearly represent the phase your child is in and the progression of their abilities. Perhaps you'll want to limit yourself to one from each month. After several years of collecting small mementos, you can turn the contents of this box into an album.

Making Scrapbooks

After you've reviewed and organized all of your photos, choose your favorites for incorporation into your photo album or scrapbook. Choose an actual album or scrapbook that conveys a specific theme, such as family vacations, holidays, family memories, or childhood. After you've decided which album to begin with, determine the sequence of the album—chronological, by themes, or by events.

The number of photographs you can get on a page will depend on the page size, the size of the photographs, and how much you crop the background of the photographs. You can, of course, be creative and overlap your photographs.

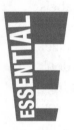

Scrapbooking.com (*www.scrapbooking.com*) and Scrapbook-Tips.com (*www.scrapbook-tips.com*) offer countless ideas for creating a highly personalized scrapbook with your photographs and other memorabilia.

When you begin to place your photos in scrapbooks, take care to purchase only albums with acid-free pages that won't damage your photos. If you do use a glue stick, use only glue sticks that are designed for photographs. Also, you can attach newspaper clippings to the pages of your album with a similar washable, nontoxic glue stick. Plastic photo sleeves are ideal for putting photos into albums quickly and for quick, safe removal.

Converting to Digital Photos

The digital revolution is one of the greatest things that has happened to photo hoarders (and those who live with them). Instead of stacks and stacks of loose, unidentifiable photos, you can now store all of your photos on your computer and only print those you love.

In addition to taking digital photos, you can also convert your old photos to a digital system. You can use a scanner to scan your existing photos to create high-resolution electronic files on your computer's hard drive, on

Zip disks, or on writable CD-ROMs. The Hewlett-Packard Photosmart photo scanner, for example, is relatively inexpensive and allows you to scan photos, negatives, or slides using any PC-based personal computer. When you want to develop photos, you can use an online service or have them developed at your regular retail developer.

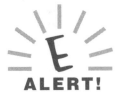

Save time now by immediately deleting photos from your camera—any photo that is out of focus can be trashed. Also, if you take a series of photos of a place or person, just choose your favorite and delete the rest. On a digital camera, there is no waste.

Many of these services also offer the option of creating photo books or calendars. These photo books can make a great gift for friends and family, and they provide a quick, easy way to create albums with the click of your mouse.

Back Up all Digital Images

Although most people have heard that digital images should be backed up, few people actually create backup files. If your entire archive of images is dependant upon your computer, however, you are in a vulnerable position. Computers can be destroyed in an instant by fire, flood, lightning, or hard-drive failure, and with the loss of your computer, you could easily lose a lifetime of photographs. An easy backup method is to create CDs with your images and store them in a different part of your home. There are a variety of ways to create reliable backups for your files and computers. To learn more about creating backups, see Chapter 5, which covers the home office.

Whether you're creating back-up for your photographs or preparing your home for guests, every bit of planning helps. By taking steps to organize and plan for your guests, you can create an environment that is restful for them and peaceful for you. No matter where your guests sleep, you can make them feel comfortable by paying attention to small details and adding comforting touches to their sleeping space. When it comes to guests, a little bit of thoughtfulness in advance goes a long way.

Chapter 13

Skeletons in the Closet

Because closets offer concealment, it can be tempting to stuff them full with mismatched items. What goes in, of course, must come out. But it often doesn't come out quite as one might hope—instead of an organized collection of board games, you open the closet door only to have an avalanche of Monopoly money and hotels come crashing down on your head. This chapter offers practical solutions for ordering your closets—and better caring for the items in there—one closet at a time.

Time to Face the Closet

Okay—take a deep breath and a moment to think. You may want to make a comforting cup of coffee or tea before you proceed. Remember that you're not going to organize all your closets today. Plan to take just one step toward your goal of orderly closets.

You may want to make a list of the closets in your home that are particular hot spots. Before you head into battle, you'll need a plan. Assess the closets throughout your home—how long would it take to organize each one? Are some closets a priority? Consider how your life is affected by the different closets in your home—perhaps the chaos in your bedroom closet affects you more than the other ones.

After you decide that your closets are in need of reorganization and how long it will take to tackle each one, create a realistic schedule for your efforts. Just as you've done in other parts of your home, you'll want to create three boxes so that you can quickly sort through your belongings. Give these boxes any name you'd like, but the gist of the titles are "Give away/ Sell," "Throw away," and "Decide later."

Shun Diversions

Now is not the time for long deliberations about what to keep and what to let go of. Now is also not the time for paging through old scrapbooks, clipping your fingernails (when you finally find that clipper!), or trying clothes on to see if they still fit (hence the "Decide later" box). The reason you want to avoid these kinds of diversions is that it is easy to go astray in the process of organizing.

It might even be helpful for you to set a timer so that you know that you're working against the clock. When the timer dings, you're done for the day, no matter how much work there is still left to do. When your session is complete, don't forget to celebrate your accomplishment in some way— shoot some photos, have a cookie, a nap, or a bath—whatever it takes to make you feel great about what you've done.

Your Road Map

If you're heading into unfamiliar terrain, you're going to need a road map. This section will outline a few basic steps to help you take back your closets (and your life!). Before beginning, determine what specific purpose the newly organized closet will have—will it store your everyday wardrobe, your coats, your linens? Be sure that your plans for each closet are directly related to location—you want your possessions to be as close as possible to the area where they will be used so that pickup is not a chore.

- Empty your closet.
- Neatly lay out the contents on a nearby floor, sofa, or bed.
- Decide which items taken out of the unorganized closet actually belong there and which items should be stored elsewhere.
- Eliminate or discard anything that's damaged, outdated, not your style, or the wrong size.

Planning Your Closets' Uses

After you discard what you no longer need from your closets, consider whether you'll eventually replace those items. For example, if you discard work clothes that are no longer in style or that no longer fit, will you buy new ones in the near future to replace them? If so, make sure you allocate room in your closet for these new purchases. The ideal with closet organization is not to come up with every smart storage solution you can, but to let go of items so that you have some empty closet space. This way, as your needs grow, your closets will "expand" to incorporate new items instead of becoming cluttered and unusable.

Although you're seeking to pare down, you'll still want to think in terms of efficient storage. Evaluate the contents of the closet and determine the best way to actually store your belongings. For example, would additional shelves, rods, or drawers provide needed space? Would these storage components make your items more visible and increase your efficiency?

Most basic closets are equipped with a single rod for hanging clothing. The height of most closets, however, allows for at least two rods, which could double the amount of space you can use to hang garments. In addition, you can use specially designed hangers to increase the number of garments you can hang in a limited amount of space.

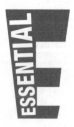

Keep your most-used items visible and easily accessible. Mary Lou Andre, president of Organization By Design, says, "We wear twenty percent of our wardrobes eighty percent of the time." To utilize the wardrobe pieces you have, she recommends assembling complete outfits, including accessories, and storing each on a single, sturdy hanger.

Plan to sort your hanging items by type or category. For example, divide up suits so that all jackets are together, all skirts are together, and so on. Sort within each category by color and/or fabric type. This can help you to create new outfit combinations by mixing and matching garments. You can divide your wardrobe into further categories—shirts, skirts, pants, jackets, suits, turtlenecks, sweaters, athletic apparel, T-shirts, jeans, and so on. You can also sort your clothing by season.

Considering Closet Organizers

Closet organizers and specialized hangers are inexpensive items that can improve the functionality of your closets. Several types of organizers fit easily into any closet.

To determine how much room you have for closet organizers (discussed in the following section), carefully measure the empty closet. Round each measurement to an eighth of an inch, taking the time to be as accurate as possible. Be sure to write the measurements down as you take them, and check your work twice.

When measuring a reach-in closet, determine the width of the closet by measuring the inside space between the two sidewalls, determine the height by measuring from the floor to the ceiling, and determine the depth by measuring the distance between the inside surface of the face wall or door and the back wall.

To measure a walk-in closet, measure the width of each wall, determine the closet's height by measuring from floor to ceiling, determine the width of the doorway by measuring the distance from frame to frame, and measure the height of the doorway, too.

General Organizers

Visit any linen superstore or check out almost any catalog or Web site that features closet organizational products and you'll find a wide selection of closet organizers. These component-based storage systems allow you to customize the inside of your closets without the high cost of hiring a professional to do it. After you've measured your available closet space and know exactly what you want to store in your closet, you can design a closet-storage system by mixing and matching modules.

Shelves and Shelf Dividers

Shelves provide you with a place to put all of the things that would otherwise go on the floor or in a dresser drawer. Preassembled stackable shelves are one option. They're available in a variety of sizes and can be customized to fit the dimensions of your closet. You can purchase closet shelving at most home-improvement or hardware stores.

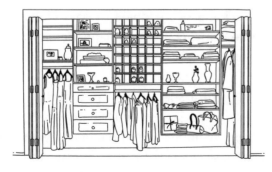

A closet organizer can inspire you to keep clutter at bay.

Shelf dividers separate your shelf into small sections that you can use for a stack of sweaters or a stash of purses, without having them tumble over or get creased or scratched. Keep in mind, however, that it can be a bit of a headache to keep these items orderly. If you've ever grabbed a neatly folded sweater from the bottom of similar stack at a retail store, you know how easily these systems disintegrate into chaos. Other divider systems organize socks, hosiery, jewelry, and folded linens.

Baskets

Ventilated baskets serve practically any purpose you can name. Removable laundry baskets in closets serve as portable hampers. Baskets in kids' closets double as portable toy bins. Mudroom baskets provide ample storage for gloves, hats, and sports gear, letting damp outerwear breathe and dry.

Canvas Wardrobe Storage

For storing off-season clothing, canvas wardrobe-storage systems can be ideal. Hanging garment bags, hanging canvas shelves for sweaters, hanging folding drawers for small items such as scarves or socks, bedding bags for storing blankets and other large items, and shoe holders are all available. You can mix and match pieces to create a customized and organized closet. You could also purchase nylon clothing protectors that offer clear, heavy-gauge vinyl windows.

Clothes Hangers

When organizing any clothing closet, you want to purchase a variety of clothes hangers. Large wooden hangers are ideal for heavy clothes such as coats. They will also help these items retain their shape. Before you decide which types of hangers are best for you, purge all bent and out-of-shape metal hangers.

Suit hangers are designed with a special pant rod so that the single hanger neatly holds both pants and a jacket. Cedar hangers absorb moisture and discourage pests (such as moths) from damaging your clothing. Collapsible, multi-tiered hangers save space by allowing you to hang multiple garments in one small area.

Shoe Racks

To improve the organization of your clothing closet, invest in a sturdy shoe rack. If you're stuck with a small closet, you might purchase a hanging shoe rack that you can attach to the back of the closet door. Most stores also sell shoe bags with pouches that you can attach to the wall of your closet. Keep in mind that the pouches built into some shoe racks can also be used to store scarves or belts. Make sure the pouches are transparent so that you can see exactly what's inside them. When storing expensive shoes, consider investing in shoetrees, devices that you place within each shoe to preserve its shape. Cedar shoetrees also absorb moisture and odors.

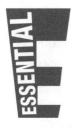

Victoria Moran says, "Cleaning your closets can be like sending your soul to a spa. As you discard the worn-out, the worthless, and the size 5 jeans that haven't fit in decades, you discard ways of thinking that no longer fit either . . . Just clean your closet. Your mind will respond."

Another possibility is a compact shoe rack that sits on the floor of your closet. These can be sloped, allowing for a better view of your shoes. As you organize your closets, strive to make everything that you use each day more visible—otherwise, you might be consistently late because of the time and effort involved with tracking down clothes that match and are clean and unwrinkled. The ideal to strive for is that everything be orderly and everything be easy to see. Every morning you want to be able to spot your clothes immediately upon opening your closet door.

Tie and Belt Racks

Although ties and belts are loose items, you can still organize and display them in your closet. Special holders or storage tacks for neckties and belts can be attached to a closet wall or door, or in some cases can be hung from the closet's rod. Some racks also slide out when you need them and tuck away when you don't. Be sure to store tie racks close to dress shirts so that coordinating outfits is easy. Pegs with nubbed tips keep ties in place and prevent wrinkling.

Jewelry Organizers

Jewelry organizers, which are often felt-lined, keep your valuable and delicate possessions cushioned and protected. In some cases, a top tray slides and lifts out, giving you two layers of storage in a single drawer. Combinations of large and small compartments work for different types and styles of jewelry and accessories.

Building Your Own Closets

After you've taken inventory of what will be stored in your closet and carefully measured the closet space you have available, you can choose to purchase prefabricated closet organizers, shelves, drawers, rods, and other organizational accessories. Most of these accessories are designed to fit standard-sized closet spaces. The trick, however, is determining in advance what closet-organizing accessories you want to implement into your closet. This means deciding what types of shelves, drawers, shoe racks, hooks, specialty hangers, and lighting you require (see the preceding section).

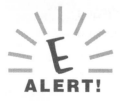

ALERT!

Although building a custom closet organizer is ideal for those who are handy with tools, if you're a novice you might want to stick with prefabricated closet organizers so that you don't become overwhelmed. Keep in mind as well that if you have to purchase costly tools, you most likely won't save money with the build-it-yourself route.

If you're handy with tools, you can build your own closet organizers from scratch. This means you'll build your organizer directly into the closet space and attached to the floor, walls, and/or ceiling. It will be custom-built to fit the exact dimensions of your closet. Custom-designing a closet is a time-consuming and risky project. A small error in measurement or calculation can cost you in terms of hours and dollars. If you've ever had to assemble a piece of furniture, you know how much longer these kinds of projects can take than you might originally anticipate.

If you're making the decision to embark on this project, you want to ensure that the end result is functional and creates the exact storage environment you need. As you begin planning what your closet will look like and how you will organize it, answer the following questions:

- Based on the appearance and organization of your closet now, what can you change to make it more organized and functional?
- Is the space currently being used efficiently?
- Is there enough room to install drawers and/or cabinets with doors that open and close?
- Do you need more shelf space, hanging space, and/or drawers in the closet? If so, how will you utilize this space?
- Can you get by using specialty hangers as opposed to doing construction and installing a customized closet organizer?
- Is the floor space and door space being utilized right now, or are shoes and other items stored inefficiently?

Hardware superstores sell do-it-yourself closet organizers, which include most of the materials you'll need to customize your closet. Just be sure that the kit you buy fits the closet you have in mind. In addition, some of the tools you'll need to install prefabricated closet organizers include a Phillips-head screwdriver (a power screwdriver is even better), hammer, stud finder, level, tape measure, circular saw or fine-tooth saw, and pipe cutter or hacksaw.

Alternative Storage Areas

Be creative about storage—there may be many places in your home where you can store seasonal items. Perhaps you have an empty crawlspace in your bedroom closet or a large guest bed that could accommodate some under-bed storage. A word of warning: when you're exploring alternative solutions, be extremely conscious of what you're storing and what type of special precautions you need to take to ensure the safety of what's being stored.

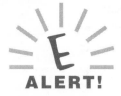

ALERT!

If you need to store clothing in a basement or attic where climate, mold, and moths may be a concern, be sure to use sturdy plastic bins instead of cardboard. Especially in a basement, you'll want to keep all items off the floor just in case a flood occurs.

Looking around your home, you'll probably find several ideal places for storing out-of-season clothing, linens, towels, bedding, and other items. For example, you might purchase an armoire for out-of-season items or even as an alternative to a closet. Wardrobes and armoires have been used as closets for centuries. Most high-end furniture stores sell various styles of armoires. You might also consider purchasing a chest that can act as a nightstand but also be used to store linens.

Maintaining Your Closets

After you've organized your closets, be sure to take a moment to revel in the glory of being able to find things quickly. Enjoy the sight of your floor and walls behind your clothes if you haven't been able to glimpse them for a while. You might even want to invite a friend over to show her your newly organized closets. You've accomplished something significant that will increase your efficiency and help you feel more at ease in your home. Allow yourself to enjoy the fruits of your labor.

The next step is a little harder than the first—you're going to want to take measures to keep your closets looking as nice as they do today. You'll probably find that your inclination is to backslide into your old ways. In fact, within a few days you might be dismayed to see your organized closets beginning to regain their former chaos. This doesn't necessarily mean that all your efforts have failed. It takes time—experts say at least twenty days—to create a new habit. If you seek to become more aware of the patterns that create the chaos, you'll be better able to change them.

Of course, it's not realistic to think that your closet will always stay perfect—and they don't need to. But if you did a good job setting up a system of organization, then you should find that your closets are more user-friendly than they were before. Keeping things neat should take less effort now. If you find kinks in your system along the way, feel free to make adjustments. Change labels on containers, reorganize clothing or shoes, and do whatever it takes to find what works for you. You'll get it right in time.

Chapter 14

Laundry Organization

Many people think of laundry as a chore that is to be avoided at all costs. But if you can organize your laundry room in a way that is visually appealing and functional, laundry day doesn't have to cause groans. This chapter has tips for organizing your laundry area and simplifying the laundering process, as well as advice about how to get tough stains out of clothing.

14

Neglected Laundry

Life is often such a whirlwind that it can be a challenge to slow down and give laundry the attention it deserves. And when we're unable to be attentive to each stage of the process, we're more likely to suffer from laundry chaos. The FlyLady compares laundry to a neglected child that turns up everywhere: "You can catch it hanging out in unsavory places: mildewed in hampers; stinky and soured in washers for days; cold and wrinkled in dryers; wadded up in baskets stashed beside beds; or folded nice and neat and left abandoned in the laundry room."

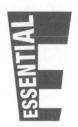

Writer Kathleen Norris has learned over the years to love doing laundry. She writes: "Hanging up wet clothes gives me time alone under the sky to think . . . and gathering the clean clothes in, smelling the sunlight on them, is victory."

Doing the laundry doesn't have to be burdensome, though. Nor does it need to consume the entire day. There are things that you can do to make this task feel more pleasant. First of all, think about the space where you do laundry. If you are lucky enough to have your own washer and dryer, there are ways that you can arrange the space to increase your efficiency. The next section outlines a few important ideas related to your laundry area.

Organizing Your Laundry Area

Wherever you locate your washer and dryer, you can probably better organize the area of your home that's dedicated to laundry. In a perfect world, a laundry area would offer the following:

- Ample space for a full-sized washer and dryer (remember to leave at least a few inches between each of these appliances and the nearby walls)

- Shelving or cabinets to store detergents and fabric softeners (the room will look less cluttered if you utilize cabinets with doors, so items can be stored out of sight)
- Space for keeping laundry baskets or hampers of dirty clothing
- An area for ironing, steaming, and folding clean clothes
- An area to hang wet clothing that needs to be line-dried
- Storage for hangers and/or a place to hang garments
- A sink for hand-washing garments
- A wastebasket
- A television, radio, and/or telephone with a speaker option to occupy your mind while you fold and iron
- Ample lighting, so you can separate different-colored clothing, identify badly stained garments for special treatment, and read the handling instructions printed on the small labels of some garments
- Temperature control, because if the laundry area gets too cold (especially in a basement), the water pipes could freeze; if the room is too hot, it will be unbearable to work in the room

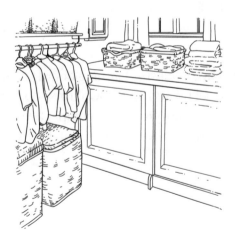

Even a closet-sized laundry room can be functional and attractive.

Unless you live in a large house or have allocated a section of your basement to accommodate all of the above-listed needs for space, chances are you'll have to improvise. Most people do, anyway. Perhaps you want to set up a laundry line outside (if your local climate is appropriate for this), or you may even want to install a retractable line above your bathtub.

One of the most important things to keep in mind when organizing your laundry area is that you want your detergents and fabric softener to be within arm's reach of the washer and dryer. Ideally, the flooring beneath your washer and dryer will be waterproof, should a flood occur. You'll also want to place an overflow container under the washer to prevent water from escaping the immediate area, should the washer overflow or leak.

Hampers

While some people have large rooms devoted to laundry, others make do with a small alcove in the bathroom or a closet. For those who must pack a lot of laundry into a small space, it is critical to think of ways to simplify the space so that everything you need is stored in way that is compact, efficient, and attractive.

If your laundry room is in a busy part of the house—or in a hallway, bathroom, or alcove—you might want to invest in a hamper that will conceal your dirty laundry. If you purchase a triple hamper—with a bin for white, light colors and dark ones—then you can simplify your life by sorting the items before they go into the hamper.

Ironing Boards

Although many people like to have a full-sized ironing board, it can take up a lot of space and be a hassle to set up and take down if you do not have a stand-alone laundry room. If your laundry space is compact, you might purchase an ironing board that comes in its own cabinet, can fold out when needed, and then be neatly concealed.

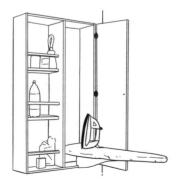

A fold-away ironing board is a clever solution for small laundry rooms.

Consider Cabinets

Another great addition to any laundry space is some cabinetry above the washer and dryer. This will allow you to store your detergent and laundry supplies out of sight, and will also afford you some useful storage for linens, towels, and other items. If the cabinetry is directly above your washer and dryer, then extra blankets, sheets and towels can simply be folded there and tucked directly into these cabinets. Be sure that there is a decent gap—at least two feet—between your appliances and the cabinets so that you have easy access to top loading machines and so that the contents of your cabinets are not exposed to too much heat or humidity.

Another benefit of cabinets—especially when a laundry area is part of another room or located in a hallway or closet—is that cabinetry can allow for a cohesive look in an area that might otherwise look thrown together. Cabinetry can distinguish the space that is used for laundry in a way that is both decorative and functional.

Flat Surfaces

Now that laundry rooms are so often small and tucked away, it can sometimes be a challenge to find a flat surface for folding clothes. If you can integrate a secondhand table or a countertop into your laundry area, this will facilitate the folding process. Think in terms of comfort as well—if you think that you'll want to sit while folding, put a comfortable chair beside the table. Make sure that you have a radio or television nearby as well, to decrease the monotony of folding your clothes.

You'll also want to be aware of lighting in this area—you'll enjoy being in there if it is adequate but not overbearing. Few people want to work happily under the glare of fluorescents. Remember that lighting can set the mood of a room, and ideally, your laundry area will be inviting and warm so that you'll actually want to spend time there. Changing the lighting doesn't have to cost much, either. Sometimes the simple addition of a floor lamp that glows instead of glares can transform the feel of the room.

Bring In Some Beauty

Who said that a laundry area has to be ugly? Especially if your laundry area is in the basement or another part of your home that does not receive much natural light, consider painting the walls a cheering color. Hang artwork or photographs that you enjoy looking at near your washer and dryer. These small touches can increase the human element of a space that is more typically dominated by machines.

Although cabinets can be functional and beautiful, they may be out of your price range. If this is the case, you can use baskets instead. A few square baskets on a shelf above the washer and dyer can be useful for keeping detergents and fabric softeners in order, and they can also add some texture and visual appeal to the area.

Everyone develops a personalized system for doing laundry. The layout and design of your laundry facilities should complement your work habits in order to make this task as stress-free and easy as possible.

Simplifying the Process

When was the last time you did several loads of laundry, wound up with missing socks, had the dye from a new pair of jeans run all over your other clothes, and then ended up with a wrinkled mess after everything came out of the dryer? Everyone has had these laundry nightmares happen, but virtually all laundry disasters and mishaps can be avoided by taking an organized approach to cleaning your clothes.

Too Much Laundry?

While working out how to best do the laundry, think about the amount of laundry you do every week. Is there any way that you can decrease your load? Do you sometimes wash clothing that isn't really dirty or linens that could be used for a few more days?

In *Simplify Your Life*, Elaine St. James suggests that while automatic washers and dryers greatly simplify the process of laundering clothing, modern Americans may be spending just as much time doing laundry as they were fifty years ago. While modern conveniences have the potential to ease our backs and make the work less labor intensive, they may not actually be reducing the amount of time we spend actually laundering our clothes.

How could this be? Because of the great ease with which clothing can be washed, many people wash their clothes far too frequently. The frenzied pace of contemporary life can sometimes cause the illusion that it is actually easier to toss a once-worn shirt into the hamper than it is to take a moment and neatly fold the shirt and place it back in a drawer or closet. The contemporary obsession with cleanliness may also add to the myth that a shirt or pants worn once is somehow "contaminated" and must be washed immediately.

Elaine St. James, however, points out that this attitude is a great departure from the practices fifty years ago, when the effort involved in laundry dictated that all family members be more careful about clothes. She writes, "In the old days, for example, Grandpa would put on a clean shirt on Monday and after wearing it carefully through the week, it would go into the clothes hamper for Grandma to take care of on wash day. Now, we think nothing of wearing two or three shirts a day, one for exercise, one for work, one for casual wear, and throwing them into the laundry."

The problem with clothing also extends to linens, according to St. James. Many people actually use a fresh towel and washcloth every single day, but this luxury can be costly in the long run. Not only does running the washer use water and energy, but it requires the vigilant efforts of a laundress. If each member of the family can reduce the amount of clothing and linens placed in the hamper each week, then the effort involved in laundering can be greatly reduced.

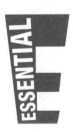

Elaine St. James urges her readers to try to limit the amount of time spent doing laundry to just one load per person per week. If family members know that only so much can be cleaned, they are likely to be more discriminating about what gets tossed into the hamper, easing the burden of the primary laundry caretaker.

Making Your Wardrobe Work for You

If you find that you consistently don't want to do laundry, try to get to the heart of the problem. Many times, resistance to doing laundry is related to problems in other parts of the house. If you've had a chance to decrease the amount of clothing in your closets and drawers, for example, you might find that you feel better equipped to do your laundry. If the drawers and closets feel overwhelming, you might be inclined to procrastinate on the final step of putting laundry away.

If this is your situation, take a break from organizing your laundry area and head back to the bedroom. Try to purge items out of a few drawers and see if a little extra space makes a difference in how you feel about putting clothing away. Drawers and closets that are packed too full are not only confusing to navigate early in the morning when you're trying to get ready for work, they also tend to leave clothes looking wrinkly and forgotten.

If you feel a sense of despair related to the idea of neatly folding your clothes, it might be related to the thought that no matter how gingerly you care for your clothes in the laundry area, they are still bound to get all wrinkled as soon as they hit the drawers. Conquer this defeating feeling by tackling the drawers and closets that are the root of the problem.

Think "Laundry Day" while Shopping

Another way to simplify your laundry is to resist impulse purchases. When shopping for clothes, don't just consider the aesthetic appeal of an item. Think also about the effort involved in cleaning it. Elaine St. James believes that life can be greatly simplified if you refuse to purchase clothing that needs to be dry-cleaned.

In certain professions, a dry-clean-only suit may be required, but for those who have the opportunity to dress more casually, eliminating dry-clean-only items from a wardrobe can reduce the hassle and cost of maintaining your clothes.

Elaine St. James also encourages people to simplify their lives by purchasing clothing that can be mixed and matched so that you don't always have to be laundering or searching for that one pair of pants that matches that one shirt. If you're really serious about simplifying your life (and you don't mind a little monotony in your wardrobe), purchase multiple pieces that are similar or the same. If you find a pair of argyle socks that you love, for example, buy four pairs so you don't have to waste precious time hunting down that one lone sock.

In *Simplify Your Life,* Elaine St. James has suggestions for women to help build a simple wardrobe. She has taken the principles of male wardrobes and adapted them to feminine standards:

- Pick a simple, classic style that looks good on you and then stick with it. Forever.
- Build combinations of outfits that work as a uniform: two or three jackets of the same or similar style but in different, muted shades, with two or three sets of the same or similarly styled skirts and/or slacks in different muted shades, and a few coordinating shirts, blouses, and tops. Each item should go with every other item.
- Remember that men, for the most part, don't wear jewelry, don't carry purses, and wear only one heel height.

These suggestions may feel a little austere, especially if you are a person who loves color and variety. You can adapt the basic concept, however, to any fashion sensibility. These are not hard and fast rules, but simply one path toward creating a simpler wardrobe.

Laundering and Ironing Your Clothes

Most clothing these days use colorfast dyes. This means that when they're washed, the colors don't run. Over time, however, if not properly taken care of, the color of fabrics will fade. Likewise, most clothing made from cotton comes preshrunk. This means that they can be placed in the dryer and not shrink. There are, however, many exceptions to these rules, so be sure to read the labels on each garment carefully before washing it for the first time.

The following are the basic steps involved in successfully washing a load of laundry using a traditional washer and dryer with off-the-shelf detergent:

- Read the care labels on each garment and follow the directions.
- Separate your clothing by color and fabric types, washing like items together.

- Empty all pockets!
- Turn down the cuffs of pants and shirts.
- Turn jeans inside out to reduce fading.
- Close all zippers, snaps, and hooks.
- On the washing machine, set the load size.
- Select the cycle type on the washer.
- Choose the appropriate water temperature on the washer (hot, warm, or cold).
- Determine the best laundry detergent, fabric softener, and bleach for the job, and then mix the appropriate amount into the washer when the directions on the detergent say to do so.
- Deal with badly stained clothing separately. This may involve using a special detergent and/or allowing the stained garment to soak before putting it through a normal wash.
- When the washer cycle is complete, remove the garments promptly. Place each garment in the dryer (if appropriate), keeping in mind that some types of garments need to be line dried and shouldn't be exposed to the high temperature of a dryer.
- To minimize wrinkling, as soon as the dryer finishes, remove the garments immediately. You may then choose to iron certain garments to completely eliminate wrinkles.

Stain-Removal Strategies

Stains are almost impossible to avoid if you live a normal lifestyle, especially if you have kids. Food, drinks, dirt, blood, grass, ink, motor oils, grease, makeup, wine, rust, chewing gum, nail polish, perspiration, and deodorants and antiperspirants are all common causes of stains you'll have to contend with sooner or later. The good news is that if you approach each stain in an organized and calm manner, you should be able to make it disappear with relative ease.

Based on the type of stain and its severity, you may choose to have a garment professionally cleaned. You can also try pretreating, presoaking, bleaching, or prewashing the garment, depending on the type of fabric and what caused the stain. Washing the stained garment in the appropriate water temperature and using the strongest possible detergent or stain remover will also help your battle against even the toughest of stains.

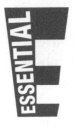

In the vintage book *Heloise's Housekeeping Hints*, she writes: "Try cutting your amount of soap in half! Overuse of soap is a common mistake among many homemakers . . . Too much soap causes soap film. If you cut the soap in half and the water still feels slippery, then you have been using too much soap."

As soon as a stain is created, take these steps:

- Sponge stains promptly with cool water to prevent the stain from setting.
- Always test your stain-removal agent on a hidden part of the garment first, to check for colorfastness.
- Before laundering, pretreat stained articles with a liquid detergent. Remember, washing and drying without any pretreatment can set some stains.
- Air-dry treated and washed items. Some residual stains are not visible when wet, and heat from the dryer could set them, making them tougher or impossible to get rid of.
- Follow all safety precautions on stain-removal product labels.
- Many stains will decrease if you apply undiluted liquid laundry detergent (such as Liquid Tide with Bleach Alternative), undiluted liquid dishwashing detergent (such as Dawn), or suds from an Ivory soap bar directly on the stained area. Launder immediately.
- For deep-set soils, old stains, extensive staining, or protein stains such as blood, grass, or urine, presoak the garment. For a maximum of thirty minutes, soak stained items in a plastic bucket or laundry tub with the warmest water safe for the fabric and a good heavy-duty laundry detergent. Bleach-sensitive stains, such as fruit juice or drink mixes, should be rinsed in cold water, and then washed with a nonchlorine bleach product. If stains remain, colorfast items may

be laundered with colorfast bleach, and bleachable items may be laundered with chlorine bleach.

Ironing

Set up the ironing board at the right height, appropriate to whether you're sitting or standing. You should be able to place your hand on the board without bending your arm (extended downward) or your back. Adjusting the ironing board to the correct height will reduce muscle fatigue.

Be sure to correctly adjust the temperature of your iron prior to getting started. Begin by consulting labels for manufacturers' suggestions, especially when ironing dry clothes. For example, when ironing blended fabrics, use the setting for the lowest-temperature fabric in the blend. Most fabrics can be ironed using the steam setting.

Start ironing each garment in the middle and work your way outward. There's no need to press too hard, especially when using steam.

Be sure to use extra care with certain types of fabrics. For example, all silks should be ironed on the reverse side. Cultivated silks should be ironed when evenly damp, but should not be sprayed because they may spot; raw silks should be ironed when dry. Velvet, acrylics, corduroy, embroidered pieces, and synthetic leathers should also be pressed from the reverse side with a clean towel or blanket on the ironing board. This will prevent these materials from ending up with an unwanted sheen.

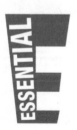

Whenever you're ironing clothes with unique fabrics, save yourself time by sorting the garments and then starting with synthetics that call for the coolest settings. By working your way up to high-temperature cottons, you'll avoid scorching and having to wait for your iron to cool down, which takes a lot longer than heating up.

When using the heat of an iron, more is not always better. Be sure to use the right temperature for each of your garments. An overheated iron is the quickest way to make your clothes go from clean to crispy. Synthetics and silks react best to low or medium temperatures. Cottons and linens react best to the iron's highest temperatures. Wools respond best to medium or high.

Putting Clothes Away

Putting clothes away can be a hassle, but recently, professional home organizers have begun to advocate an interesting approach to putting clothing away. Instead of separating your socks, slacks, and shirts into neat little piles, they advise assembling outfits and then storing entire outfits on hangers or in your drawers. This small step can add ease to your mornings, because you no longer have to look for the skirt that goes with a particular shirt. This approach is also very helpful for children, because sometimes assembling outfits that actually match can be a challenge for them. But if you assemble outfits for them and place similar items together in their drawers, your children will be able to feel independent when they "pick" their own outfit, without actually exercising the kind of independence that will make you cringe when they come out of their rooms.

Like every room in the house, the laundry area is full of challenges, but these challenges can become opportunities. As you become more attuned to bringing order, harmony, and functionality to this part of your life, you might find that the dread associated with doing laundry will decrease. Victoria Moran's book *Shelter for the Spirit* says that we often dislike monotonous tasks such as cleaning or laundry simply because we feel that they are mindless and perhaps "beneath us." But these concrete tasks are a very real way to care for those who surround us.

After you have rearranged and decorated your laundry area to make it more efficient and appealing, you might find the groans come less often.

Chapter 15

Dark Places: Attics and Basements

The attic and basement tend to attract clutter because it can be so simple to stash items in these large, empty spaces. You might often be tempted to think "Out of sight, out of mind"—yet all that clutter above and below can weigh on you. It can be a fire hazard as well as a haven for unwanted pests. This chapter explores ways to make organizing the attic and basement efficient—and possibly even fun!

15

Tackling Your Basement

Before you start to panic, take a deep breath and remind yourself that you don't have to organize these areas in a single afternoon—nor should you take on this task all by yourself. In Julie Morgenstern's book *Organizing from the Inside Out*, she writes that basements should be family projects if you want to enjoy them over the long haul. Everyone should have something invested in keeping that area in order. Prior to beginning to organize the basement, she suggests that you have a family meeting so that each member can consider what he might gain through a more organized basement or attic.

The chaos in the attic or basement could be preventing your family from enjoying the space to the fullest. Not only does chaos make it harder to retrieve items when you need them, it can also prevent your family from spreading into these parts of the house. Could your basement or attic provide a play room for small children or an entertainment area for older ones? If so, talk that up! You're likely to get more cooperation from your children if they know that there is something in this project for them.

Finding a Place for Everything

One of the great traps of the basement is that it can be easy to stash items away without really paying attention to how items are grouped. This can be especially troublesome if several members of the family are doing the same thing. Pretty soon, your basement or attic becomes a jungle that nobody wants to navigate.

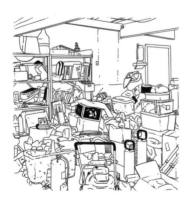

A cluttered basement.

Clutter-Bust

As in every part of your home, you'll want to try to crack down on clutter in these areas. The basement will seem much more manageable after you've gotten rid of the excess. If members of your family are open to getting rid of some of the items in your basement, you might consider assigning each family member the task of finding five or ten items to give away. You could even make it a race against each other or against the clock. If you're all working together, the project can move at a steady clip. That said, one rule stands: nobody is allowed to get rid of other people's possessions. The game can turn ugly pretty fast if family members are insensitive in this regard. Make sure all of the rules are clear from the beginning.

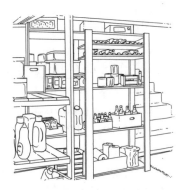

An organized basement.

Finding a Home for Your Possessions

Usually basements and attics are not very well-planned spaces. As you consider the items in your basement, it might be helpful to begin to think of them in terms of groupings—like items, such as sports equipment, wrapping paper and ribbons, or toys can be placed together so that they will be easier to find. Consider drawing a diagram of how and where you'd like items to be stored.

As you begin to organize your possessions into groupings, think about what types of storage might work. Sometimes you might be able to increase storage capacity by changing the arrangement of the storage devices you already own. Bookshelves that are placed perpendicular to the wall, for example, can increase storage and can help differentiate the space.

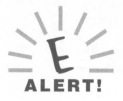

ALERT!

Even if you have ample lighting in your basement, keep a high-intensity, battery-powered flashlight near the entrance. If you lose power, you might need to access your fuse box, hot water heater, or furnace. Check the flashlight batteries monthly.

As you consider different storage zones, organize your belongings according to category, such as "holidays," "sports," "memorabilia," and so on. There are some items that might be in your attic or basement for purely sentimental reasons. If you need to hold on to these items, there are a few things you could do to reduce the physical space they consume.

You can create a memorabilia box for each family member. Whatever the size of the box, you would seek to limit the amount of items saved to what you could fit in that box. Ideally, the box would be plastic to protect fragile paper or photographs. While it can be worthwhile to hold on to items of sentimental value, it's best to put some kind of system into place that will force you to be selective. Another idea is to take a picture of items that have sentimental value but you know will never have a place in your home. Instead of holding on to the actual item, you can hold on to the photo (or better yet—you can store the image on your computer). This compromise will allow you to retain a link to the memory or person that the item represents without using precious storage.

Here are some guidelines for storing items:

- Clean, package, and/or launder the items. Items that go into storage in good condition are more apt to stay that way longer. Polish your jewelry or silver flatware before storing it.
- Categorize.
- Sort and place similar items together.
- Place items in appropriate (airtight) storage containers, which come in a variety of sizes.
- Label. Mark each carton, container, or item with a descriptive label that's easily visible. For example, "Summer Clothing," "Baby Clothing," "1998 Personal Financial Records," "Christmas Decorations," or "Winter Jackets."

- Store in such a way that your belongings can be easily found and retrieved without your having to dig through endless piles of stuff.

In any hardware store, you'll find a wide range of plastic and metal shelving units, some that are standalone units and others that need to be bolted and installed directly onto your walls. After you decide what smaller items you'll be keeping and what you will store in your basement, choose the best method for storing these smaller items, using boxes, shelving, cabinets, or perhaps a pegboard with hooks that gets mounted on a wall.

A Good Cleaning

The great thing about clearing out the basement is that now that you can see the floors and walls, you can get the dust and spiders out of there. Before you put anything back into the space, make sure that you've cleaned out the cobwebs. Otherwise, even if you've created some order, you'll probably still dread going down to the basement. Who wants to encounter spiders, dust, and grime?

To protect the items to be stored, think about what's required: cardboard boxes, airtight plastic containers, shelves, drawers, coverings (tarps), and so on. You can also store items by hanging them from the basement ceiling.

Next, install the shelving, lighting, or other organizational tools you believe are necessary. After the room is prepared, fill your basement with the items you plan to store there, starting with the largest items first. Refer to your hand-drawn diagram to figure out where things will go.

As you evaluate your storage plan, answer the following questions:

- Are the items you're storing easy to find and readily accessible?
- Are the items you're storing far enough away from your laundry area or workshop area? Is there a clear path to your working appliances, as well as ample space to work and play?
- If you have children, does your storage area provide any potential hazards? Should certain items be locked up separately?
- Have you protected your belongings against natural disasters and pests (flooding, mildew, mold, insects, and rodents)?

- Are your stored items in the way of your home's hot water heater, furnace, fuse box, washer, dryer, or any other appliances in use within the basement? Are all drains and pipes clear from any obstruction?

If you're storing plastic crates or boxes, stack them up against a wall, making sure they are stable and won't fall. Also, make sure that the labels (describing what's in each box) are facing outward and are easily readable. Place the larger and heavier boxes on the bottom, and the lighter ones above them. Items stored in boxes at the bottom of the piles should be the ones you'll need the least often. Make sure you keep flammable items away from your furnace, hot water heater, washer, dryer, and any other potential heat sources.

Seasonal Organizing

As you decide where your various items will be stored, think in terms of when they'll be used. For example, you may want to store your winter clothing in containers near your holiday decorations. Likewise, you may want to store your grill near your Fourth of July decorations and lawn furniture. If you tend to go on a family vacation every summer (and use your luggage), you may want to store your luggage near your summer items for easy access.

Your most frequently used items should receive prime storage space so they're most readily accessible any time of the year. If you also use your basement as a workshop, exercise room, or hobby area, make sure your storage area is kept separate. You can use room dividers or other methods to section off each area of your basement as needed.

Organizing Your Attic

The environment of an attic is very much like a basement: cold, dark, and damp. In most homes, however, the attic is more difficult to access. Hence, you're best off using the attic for storing only lighter or smaller items, such as off-season clothing, empty luggage, holiday decorations, empty boxes from electronics equipment (e.g., computer, DVD player, fax machine), or sports equipment.

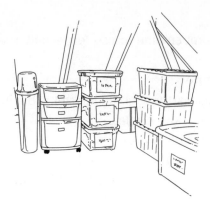

Use your attic for long-term storage solutions.

Considering Access

If you'll be using the attic as a storage area and will need to gain access to this space often, you might want to replace the basic access-panel entrance (which you may need a ladder to get to) with a pull-down staircase. Also, install a light switch or light pull-string near the entrance to the attic. You don't want to be climbing around in the dark. For information on pull-down staircases, visit any hardware or home-improvement store. You can also point your Web browser to the Louisville Ladder Web site (*www.ladderpros.com*) and click on Products—Attic Ladders.

Treat organizing your attic in almost exactly the same way you would handle the basement. In other words, know that you'll be storing your items in a non-climate-controlled environment (with potential hazards such as water, mildew, mold, insects, and/or rodents), and take the appropriate precautions. Airtight plastic storage containers are useful and economical—make sure they're clear so that you can see the contents, but don't forget to label them as well.

Tackling Clutter

Throughout the attic-organization process, be critical about items stored there. Because an attic is rarely climate controlled, items stored there can be easily damaged. You might want to ask yourself if the items up there are even needed—if you haven't thought about them for years, they might not be important enough to keep.

Here is a list of items that every home can do without:

- Old tools that don't work
- Luggage that is broken or cumbersome to use (especially if you've updated your luggage)
- Mildewed or damaged furniture
- College textbooks (in some cases, these could be useful, but in most fields the material becomes quickly obsolete)
- Old mattresses that are just collecting dust
- Appliances that no longer work or are rarely used
- Cassette tapes and VHS tapes if you only use a DVD/CD player

Be attentive to the things around you that are taking up precious space. Although it can be painful to let certain items go, it is visually thrilling to see your home with less clutter. The FlyLady says that decluttering allows your home to breathe. Keep in mind that by decluttering you may be giving your home a great gift—the gift of fresh life.

Safe Storage

Unless you're using airtight containers, don't store paper-based items, such as photos, books, or other important documents, in the attic. Videotapes and audiocassettes, as well as any type of electronic equipment, won't do well in a potentially damp environment with extreme hot or cold temperatures.

Better Uses for the Space

Begin organizing your attic space by determining how you plan to utilize this space. Decide what you want to store in your attic, and then measure the attic space carefully and make sure it's suitable for your needs. Prepare your attic for its intended purpose, eliminating potential hazards.

Using a pad of paper and your measurements, draw a rough layout of the area and determine how and where you'll be storing your various belongings. Figure out whether you'll first need to install additional shelving, lighting, flooring, or anything else to make your attic space more usable.

As you did with your basement, after you've had a chance to remove the clutter from your attic, give the space a good cleaning. This cleaning is not only useful for your sense of well-being, but it can also lead to important information. Perhaps your roof has a leak that you hadn't known about. A good cleaning can reveal water spots, squirrels' nests, and all sorts of hidden problems. After the area is cleaned out, begin arranging the items you're storing in the attic. Put items you won't need often in places where they're less readily available. As you arrange boxes and other items in the attic, make sure air vents are unobstructed. Also, if there is a ventilation fan in the attic, make sure your items are kept away from it.

Extra Living Space?

Many families wonder if their attic could expand their living space. Because most attics weren't built for this kind of use, you'll want to address the following concerns before making any remodeling plans:

- Does the attic offer ample headroom?
- After it's complete, what will the room be used for?
- Is there an easy-to-access stairway leading to the attic space?
- Are the floor joists large enough to support the added load?
- What will it cost to transform the attic into a finished room? Is the investment worth the added functionality you'll receive from the room after it's in use?

As you consider your options, speak with friends who have had similar work done. Invite contractors and architects to view the potential project and give you an assessment of feasibility and potential cost. Although a redone attic can provide valuable living space, keep in mind that this type of project can be surprisingly complicated and costly.

Public Storage Facilities

When the storage space available in your closets, basement, attic, and garage just isn't enough, you do have other options. Public storage facilities are available across the United States that provide extra storage space for a flat monthly or annual fee. Public Storage (*www.publicstorage.com*) is just one nationwide chain of public storage facilities. Public Storage manages over 1,400 self-service storage locations in eighty U.S. and Canadian cities. In addition to offering storage facilities, the company offers pick-up service, which is particularly useful for transporting large and heavy items from your home to the storage unit you rent.

To find other self-storage facilities in your area, check the Yellow Pages or point your Web browser to SelfStorageNet (*www.selfstoragenet.com*), which offers a directory of facilities, plus tips on how to maximize this type of storage space.

The storage facility provides a written agreement when you rent the space. Make sure you read this agreement carefully. Check the paperwork for your payment date and determine whether the agreement covers prorated rental periods. Also ask how and when your security deposit will be refunded.

Before You Store

If you're seriously considering self storage, there are a number of issues to consider. Keep in mind that keeping things in storage can complicate future moves, and that the cost is ongoing—you will pay fees for as long as you keep the storage. That said, if you have furniture or other items that you'd like to save for a second home or for your children, this option could make sense.

Consider the following questions as you evaluate self-storage options:

- What size units are available?
- What is the monthly/annual fee for renting the space?
- Can you rent month to month or is a long-term agreement required?
- What type of security is offered? Is there always a guard on duty?
- Are the facility and the individual storage units climate controlled?
- How much of a deposit is required?
- What are the guidelines in terms of what can and can't be stored at the facility?
- Can you obtain access to your storage unit twenty-four hours per day, 365 days per year?
- What paperwork must you sign to rent a storage unit?

Deciding Whether You Need Climate Control

As you begin to narrow down your storage options, you'll need to decide whether to use climate-controlled storage. Many people store items in basements and attics without any problem, but depending on your storage needs, climate could be an issue.

A climate-controlled space guarantees that nothing will be damaged by extreme hot or cold temperatures. This would mean that certain items, such as some electronics, as well as photographs and paper, could safely be stored.

Utilize climate-controlled storage space for items such as books, business files and records, cleaning supplies, computers, crystal and glassware, electronic equipment, fine linens and clothing, leather furniture, mattresses, musical equipment, oil paintings, paint supplies, pharmaceutical products, pianos, and retail inventory items.

Organizing Your Storage Space

After your storage unit has been rented, you'll want to carefully organize it. If you don't take the time to organize before you store, you won't be able to access the things you need in your storage.

Here are a few tips for organizing your storage:

- Lay down cardboard, pallets, or skids on the floor of your storage space.
- Create a walkway inside your storage space to allow for easier access.
- Keep items that you need to access frequently at the front of your storage space.
- Draw and label a map of where everything is located in your storage space.
- For better ventilation, leave a few inches of space between your items and the storage space's walls.
- Stack similarly sized boxes together.
- Stack heaviest items on the bottom and lighter items on the top.
- Store pictures and mirrors on their sides.
- Disassemble table legs to save space.

- Place mattresses on end so they stand straight up. You might want to have mattresses shrink-wrapped to protect against any encroachment of water or pests into your space.
- To protect against dust, cover exposed items with old blankets.
- Store sofas on end to conserve space.
- Always lock your storage space.

By taking care when you store your belongings, you'll be better able to protect your investments. Although using outside storage is expensive and really a last resort, there are situations when rented storage can be useful. It can work especially well as a temporary measure if, for instance, you'll be traveling for a year or so, or if you're moving and there will be a lag time between when you will take possession of your new home and move out of your current home.

Security Precautions for Apartment or Condo Storage

If you live in an apartment or condo, you may have access to storage space in a basement or attic; however, this space may be shared with other tenants or residents. In this situation, you can still store your belongings, but you'll need to contend with security issues and avoid storing anything extremely valuable or sentimental.

Keep It Locked

When storing items in a communal storage facility, make sure you use containers that can be locked, especially if the area or storage cubicle you have access to is not totally secure. You'll still want to use airtight containers to store belongings such as clothing, books, papers, memorabilia, and so on, but you'll also want to take additional security precautions. For example, use containers that are opaque (not clear or see-through) and don't visibly label your containers. Instead, number them and keep the list of the contents of each numbered container to yourself. If someone happens to break into the communal storage space, you don't want to make it easier for them to find valuable items to steal or damage.

Larger and Valuable Items

If you'll be storing larger items, such as sports equipment (bikes, skis, and so on), make sure you lock these items up separately. Somehow attach or bolt the locks to a wall, floor, or ceiling. Take steps to ensure that these larger and more expensive items are not readily visible to someone casually peeking into the storage facility.

When placing boxes, plastic storage containers, or other items in your basement or attic, never store them directly on the floor. Insert plastic or wooden pallets on the floor below your items. This will raise your items up slightly as a precaution against flooding. If possible, try not to store items too close to a window or washing machine to protect against water.

Safes and Safety-Deposit Boxes

For the ultimate protection of valuable or important papers, documents, jewelry, and other small belongings, you may want to invest in a safe, which can be bolted to a wall or floor, making it extremely difficult to steal. A good safe is also fireproof and waterproof. If you have just a small number of important documents, you can always rent a safe-deposit box at a local bank or financial institution.

It's Worth It!

Although tackling your basement and attic can be a daunting task, there are many hidden rewards to this kind of project. You may even be able to enlarge your home, without the cost of an addition. You'll also regain access to those things that you need and love.

And, if you are able to remove clutter and donate it charity, you'll have the opportunity to be socially and ecologically responsible. Instead of all that stuff wasting away in the dark, cobwebby corners of your basement and attic, at least some of these items could be put to use by those who need them, and others could be recycled into something useful for others to enjoy. Meanwhile, you'll have the opportunity to live in less cluttered, more streamlined space. As Leonardo da Vinci wrote, "Simplicity is the ultimate sophistication."

Chapter 16

The Great Outdoors

Sometimes, clutter spills out of the home and into the outside space. Decks, patios, and sheds often need attention to become and remain useful and attractive. As you bring order to your yard, you have an opportunity to create a serene refuge for your family—a place for play, peace, and entertaining. This chapter offers helpful information on how to fulfill the true potential of your outdoor space.

Your Deck and Patio

Deck and patio space is often at a premium, so you'll want to be careful about how you arrange the space. You'll want to make sure that any furniture you select is not too large for the existing space, and if you often have guests, you'll want to be able to add seating should the need arise. Invest in high-quality furniture because deck furniture will be exposed to the elements (even if you store it inside during the winters). Try to buy top-quality items at the end of the season when they're all on sale, or at outlet stores from manufacturers you trust. If you visit an outlet store at the end of the season, you could save as much as 70 percent on your purchase. You'll get quality furniture that will last for years to come, but you'll pay a fraction of the original cost.

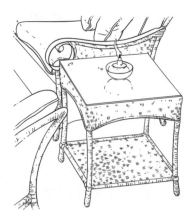

Comfortable and attractive patio furniture can add a room to your home.

Also, think in terms of comfort. If you love to sit outside and read or you'll be spending hours out there watching your kids, you'll never regret purchasing a chair that is as comfortable as your inside furniture. Many stores sell deck chairs with ottomans that have large, durable, washable weatherproof cushions that wear well over time. Investing in high-quality cushions will let you kick back and enjoy the outdoors.

One of the best ways to keep your deck and patio uncluttered is to store any items that you aren't currently using. Frequently purge items the moment they lose their value—cracked pots need not be fixed, bent rakes will do you no good in the fall. Take a ruthless approach to keeping broken things out of your yard, and you'll be better able to appreciate the beauty that thrives there. When plants die (as they inevitably will), take care of them promptly instead of watching their slow disintegration on your porch. This can be depressing for you and can compromise the beauty and freshness of your outdoor space.

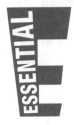

You'll want to bring cushions in to store them for the winter, but make sure that they have been cleaned and completely dried before you tuck them away. Otherwise, stains will set and mold might even intrude, making the cushions unusable. Also, be sure to store cushions in an area that is free from mold and humidity.

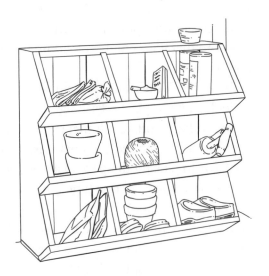

Bins provide extra storage on the patio.

Be sure to keep lawn implements in a shed or garage instead of right on the limited patio/porch space. Also, if space is tight, you might use window boxes or plant boxes along the perimeter of the porch so that you don't use up valuable space on your porch.

Consider purchasing hardy wood furnishings (benches and the like) that can provide storage on your deck. These can often be found with wheels on the bottom, which will dramatically increase their function—should you have company over, you can easily rearrange these items to make your guests comfortable.

Kids and Your Yard

A yard can be a great place for little feet and little minds to explore. Children who play outside have the opportunity for much-needed unstructured free play, while those who sit inside in front of the television are more likely to struggle with obesity.

Although having a yard is great for families with small children, these green spaces can present many challenges, especially if you've accumulated more playthings than your children know how to use. Be aggressive about purging outdoor toys when they are rarely used, and place the burden of the work on your children's shoulders. You might purchase a small wagon so that your children can easily transport their own toys outside. After an afternoon of play, make sure that your children load up the wagon and return the toys to their inside home.

If you want to keep toys in the yard, you can use a sturdy plastic toy chest that can be kept on the deck. A large plastic garbage bin can serve as great storage for bats, balls, and other sports equipment. To reduce the possibility of a yard littered with plastic toys (and kids who are too overwhelmed by the sheer number of toys to pick them up themselves), you can limit the number of toys allowed in the yard at any one time (choose a number that works for your family, such as five or ten).

You might also want to rotate toys that are kept in the bin. Many times, if toy bins are too overstuffed, kids won't remember what toys they have. Toys are quickly outgrown, and some toys never capture a kid's interest. If you purge these items, your child will be better able to see what he has. Not only will the child play more with the toys he does have, but he'll also be more likely to participate in cleanup.

In terms of play equipment in the yard—gym equipment, plastic playhouses, and the like—take note of how often they are used. If you begin to sense that your children are no longer enjoying them, look for another home for these items. These kinds of things tend to be bulky, heavy, and difficult to move. Simplify your life (and beautify your yard) by getting rid of as many of these items as you (and your children) can let go of.

Make sure that all of this equipment is still safe for use. When these items begin to break down and become warped, get rid of them quickly to protect your children's safety. Because these items are often used for climbing, jumping, and other energetic activity, you'll want to be sure that they are structurally sound. Also check with the manufacturer about appropriate ages and weights. As soon as children become too large or old, consider passing the items on to smaller children in the neighborhood.

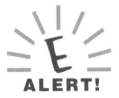

ALERT!

If your children haven't used the play equipment in the backyard for several months, ask them why. Perhaps they've begun to outgrow the items or bugs have gotten into them. Playhouses can quickly become havens for insects and litter boxes for cats. Once you uncover the problem, you can remedy the situation or get rid of the equipment.

Fire Up the Grill

The position of your grill is extremely important. If it is too close to your home or stored on a wood porch, it could present a fire hazard. You'll also want to keep it several feet away from your outside dining or sitting area. Before purchasing a grill, think about how often you will use it and where it will be stored. If you'll only use it occasionally, your best bet is probably a grill that is on wheels and can be stored in a shed or garage.

Purchasing a grill can be a confusing task because there are so many options available. Some are natural-gas powered, while others use propane gas or charcoal. Also, to lengthen the life of charcoal or smoking chips, keep them dry and raised.

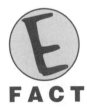

FACT

Propane gas is a fire hazard. Do not store propane tanks in your home. A shed is a better option. If storage of flammable materials is a problem, you might want a gas grill that can be installed on your deck and connected to your home's gas supply. With a direct gas line, you can fire up the grill instantly without charcoal or propane.

If you'll be grilling near children, take extra caution with matches, lighter fluid, and all flammable materials. Warn children that the grill will remain extremely hot for a long time after use. Grill tools are also often sharp and dangerous, so these should be carefully tucked away after use.

You can purchase a small, lockable storage chest to keep on your deck or patio. Inside, you can store items such as citronella candles, grilling utensils, matches and other items. If you store anything flammable in this chest, make sure to keep all cloth products and sporting equipment in another area.

Storage Sheds

It you have several bulky items that you want to keep close to your yard, consider purchasing an outdoor storage shed. An outdoor storage shed is ideal for housing a lawn mower, rakes, garden hoses, sprinklers, shovels, fertilizers, and other garden tools. These small sheds are built to withstand the elements and to provide non-climate-controlled storage inside.

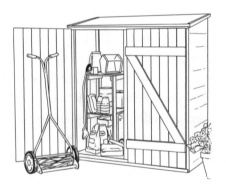

A small storage shed can keep valuable tools safe.

One of the things to keep in mind when planning for a shed is that many communities have regulations pertaining to sheds. These requirements concern such details as where a shed can and can't be located, its size, and possibly its appearance.

As you plan for a shed, think in terms of aesthetics as well as function. Sheds can be purchased in natural woods, such as cedar, which is rot-resistant (although it does require maintenance). Some materials, such as steel, are prone to rust, while aluminum is far more durable. Likewise, if you choose to purchase a shed with vinyl siding, make sure that you invest in a high-quality product so that the siding will not warp over time.

Before purchasing a shed, you'll need to answer the following questions:

- What elements and other conditions will your shed be exposed to?
- What will you be storing in your shed?
- Do the contents of your shed need to be kept in a water-free environment?
- Does the shed need to be temperature controlled?
- Will the shed require electricity?
- Based on what you need to store, how large must the shed be?
- Where on your property will the shed be installed?

Storage sheds are available in a variety of shapes, sizes, and orientations: horizontal or vertical, top or front-loading, with lifting or sliding roofs. They are generally simple to assemble and require little or no maintenance. The greatest challenge they might pose (like your garage) is the challenge of keeping the items within them organized. It can be tempting, with any space that is rarely seen, to let clutter accumulate and chaos reign. If you know that you tend to toss random items into your closets inside the house, you might want to avoid purchasing a shed, as it could present further temptations to you. To find out more about specific shed options, see Appendix A at the back of this book.

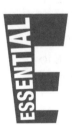

Sheds can be placed on several different types of foundations. A shed can be placed on a 3- to 4-inch bed of crushed stone. If the site is soft or you want protection from frost, use a pier foundation with pressure-treated columns on concrete footings. Sheds can also be placed on concrete or stone patios.

Because your shed is a semi-permanent structure, you'll want to take care when choosing a location for it. It must be level, and you want to be sure that the ground around the shed drains properly so that you do not flood your shed. Also, keep in mind that any door on a shed should have adequate clearance for storing your largest items, such as a lawn mower.

Organizing the Interior of Your Shed

In addition to your lawn mower, leaf blower, long-handled gardening equipment, bicycles, and other large items, you'll find that a shed is also ideal for storing smaller items such as gardening tools. Place these smaller items on shelves or in a place where they're easily accessible—make sure, for example, that you won't have to move your lawn mower every time you want to retrieve a garden tool. Keep the items you'll only use once a month in the back of the shed, where they won't be as easily accessible. As you arrange items in your shed, continually ask yourself how often you'll need access to each item and organize the space accordingly.

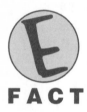

FACT

To make the most of your storage shed, you can install a pegboard or hooks along the walls. This will let you store things so that they are easy to spot and retrieve and easy to replace. Keep storage as hassle free as possible and you will be less inclined to avoid putting things in their proper locations.

Because the shed provides extra storage, be vigilant about what you place in there. You may find yourself tempted to place items in there that you will never use again, such as broken tools and cracked flower pots. Throw out things that break immediately so that you won't have the extra burden of trying to sort through them later on. Also, you'll want to be able to see all of the things in your shed so that you don't end up rushing out to the store to replace something you already own.

Caring for Your Tools

Your garden tools are costly and can rust and warp over time if they're not cared for properly. Take care to clean these tools before the winter. You can do this by running each tool under water and drying it completely, or passing the tool through a bucket of sand. You can also keep rust at bay by applying linseed oil to the tools.

Your lawn mower also needs attention at the end of summer and before winter sets in. You'll want to follow the manufacturer's instructions for cleaning the blades.

Terra cotta pots are also prone to mold. In order to prevent mold, be sure to give them a good cleaning before winter. After you've removed their contents, scrub the pots and then soak them overnight in a solution that is ½ cup bleach to a gallon of water to wipe-out mold. Be sure to rinse and dry them completely before you store them. Also, mold hates sunlight. After you've had a chance to soak and dry them, leave the empty pots in a hot, sunny corner of your deck or patio as an extra precautionary measure.

Martha Stewart suggests that you can cleverly recycle sturdy old rake heads by hanging them high on a wall of your home or storage shed. From the rake head, you can hang a variety of small garden tools. She also says that you can neatly store your hose by purchasing a large metal bucket, drilling holes in the bottom of it, and attaching this item to the side of your home— you can stash your sprinkler or different hose heads inside of the bucket.

Keeping It Low Maintenance

Especially for first-time homeowners, the work and cost involved in maintaining a lawn can often come as quite a shock. In *Simplify Your Life*, Elaine St. James suggests that if you find keeping a lawn to be burdensome, you should consider how often your lawn is used and whether grass or a lower-maintenance ground cover would work best for you. She suggests that you check with a nursery about hardy ground covers that thrive in your locale—drought-tolerant and low-maintenance ground covers such as pachysandra, dichondra, and ivy.

She also offers these tips for simplifying lawn care (if you do choose to keep your lawn):

- Make the lawn portion of your yard smaller.
- Many types of grass have an opportunity to grow healthier roots when they can grow up to 2 or 3 inches. Keep in mind that the taller the grass, the more shade is provided by each blade, thus not only will the grass weather the heat better, but less water will evaporate.

- Take care not to overwater your lawn (according to Elaine St. James, most people overwater their lawns by 40 percent). Water slowly and deeply and keep in mind that certain times of the day are far better for watering than others—to fortify your grass for the day ahead (and to reduce evaporation) water in the early morning.
- Use organic fertilizers (if you need them) and don't pick up the lawn clippings. Not only is it simpler to leave them there, but they are better used in your yard than in a landfill. These clippings actually serve as a natural fertilizer.

If your yard is small enough, you might want to purchase a manual (push) mower. These mowers are much easier to move than their bulkier gas or electric counterparts, and they never need to be charged and never run out of gas. They are ecologically friendly and they might even help tone your arms for the summer months. Keep in mind that if your mower is easy to transport from your shed or garage, then you will be more likely to use it—and less likely to let the grass get completely out of control.

Caring for Your Yard During a Drought

During a drought when water is limited, you're better off giving water to your trees rather than your lawn. Lawns are incredibly resilient and can be recovered during a moisture-rich year. Trees, however, are costly to replace and grow slowly. Trees need the moisture during the summer months to fortify them for the year ahead. If trees are treated well, they serve as natural air conditioners in the yard, providing a shady place to rest on even the hottest of days.

Pets and the Yard

While it can be a great luxury to open your back door and let the dog make his own choice about where to go, this practice can be very hard on your lawn. Dog urine is caustic for grass and will leave unsightly brown spots. One solution is to train your dog to use the same area every day, an area in which you've placed small pebbles or wood chips. This will make it easy to spot droppings that need to be removed, and will reduce harm to your greenery.

Because dogs will generally follow the scent from the day before, training them to use the same area should not be too difficult. Begin by placing the dog on a leash and taking him to the same spot every day. Praise the dog when he goes in that spot, and perhaps give him a treat. Eventually, your dog will be conditioned to go only in one area. You will have a much simpler job keeping that area clean, your lawn will be preserved, and your kids can play in the grass without worries. Another way to reduce wear and tear on the portion of a yard used by dogs is to install brick or stone pathways. These pathways add an attractive accent to the yard, and it can be easy to spot and clean droppings on them.

Get the Hose Out

Even if you've trained your dog to go only in designated areas, your dog, or a stray dog, may occasionally urinate on the grass. When this occurs, quickly get a hose and dilute the spot where the dog urinated. The water will prevent the high concentration of salt and nitrates that can be the most harmful to your grass.

Enjoying the Fruits of Your Labor

Although gardening can be some work, it is also very relaxing and rewarding in a tangible way. With a small amount of effort, you can nurture plants that are attractive and tasty. Many people think that gardens can simplify your life because they force you to focus on concrete realities. Also, instead of rushing to the store to purchase herbs or tomatoes at the last minute, you can often grow these goodies and have them available all summer (and in small containers in the kitchen all winter) for your favorite recipes.

Not only is gardening great for adults, it can help children (especially city kids) begin to understand the connection between the earth and the food consumed every day. Gardens can even inspire picky eaters to taste veggies they might otherwise shy away from, because who can reject something that they have grown and nurtured? Gardening can also help kids appreciate the seasons and experience fruits and veggies in their freshest, tastiest form. This kind of experience can leave a lasting impression on little palates.

Caring for Plants

In order to best care for your plants, you'll want to take a careful approach to how you water them. For large potted plants, a good rule of thumb is that you have given them enough water when they are difficult to move with your foot. If they easily slide across the patio, they are probably still thirsty. For window and rail boxes, water the plants just enough so that the water begins to drip out. Also, to allow for proper drainage for container plants, when placing a plant in a pot, recycle Styrofoam popcorn. Place an upside-down plastic pot inside a container, surround it with Styrofoam, and then pack soil around your plant and on top of the popcorn. This hearty soil-substitute will also make it easier for you to move your container plants, should the need arise.

A Small Space Can Still Be Productive

Even if you only have a postage-sized deck, try keeping a few herbs or plants on your deck. You can start small—grow cherry tomatoes for one season, for example, and see how manageable the work is. You can also grow strawberries (a favorite with kids) in a small container.

Try purchasing plants at a farmers' market that specializes in local, organic produce. You can talk directly to the farmers about ways to make your veggies thrive, and you can be assured that the quality of the plant is high. Also, if something does go wrong with the plants or seedlings you purchase, you can return to the farmers' market and ask additional questions about how to make your plants healthy.

Cultivate Delight

Whatever you choose to do with your own little patch of green, keep in mind that this space allows you the opportunity to create sensory delight—you can grow edibles here, nurture lovely flowers, or create a serene retreat to relax in at the end of the day. The order you bring to the outside of your home need not be as elaborate as the order you seek to cultivate inside your home, but it can certainly be nourishing to your soul and body. If you are intentional about making your yard a place that is both healthy and beautiful, you will bless your neighbors and yourself. There are millions of ways to do this in your yard. Experiment with different ideas until you're able to create the green space you desire. And whatever you do, cherish the time spent in your yard. Millions of people in urban areas around the world would relish the opportunity to have a small patch of green to call their own—a place for solitude, reflection, and transformation. As Diane Ackerman writes, "Just cultivate delight. Enjoy the sensory pleasures of the garden. That's number one." If you can cultivate delight, the rest will fall into place.

Chapter 17

The Garage and Car

All over America, garages are bursting at the seams with clutter. Many cars are relegated to driveways because of all the things stashed in the garage. Cluttered garages are costly—cars forced to sleep outside won't have the lifespan of their garage-protected counterparts. They quickly rust and are more likely to be broken into. And the clutter in your garage also complicates life because on snowy mornings, you have to be out there scraping off your car. This chapter offers ways to simplify your life by organizing your garage.

Working Through Your Garage

Because your garage is a non-climate-controlled space, you'll want to be very careful about storing items there. Certain items, such as bikes, garden tools, and lawnmowers, are hearty enough to hold up in the garage. Other items—including anything made of cloth or paper—should not be stored in the garage because of the possibility of mold and damage. Ideally, you want to store less in your garage so that the few things you do store there will be readily accessible.

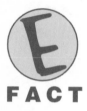

FACT

If your garage feels chaotic, know that you are not alone. Nearly 50 percent of American homeowners who were surveyed admitted that their garage was disorganized, according to the National Association of Professional Home Organizers. One-third of this group added that their garage was the messiest place in their home.

As you begin work on your garage, plan a strategy that will work for you. If you'll be working with your family or friends, create incentives—such as pizza at the end of the day—to help the work go more smoothly. Also, begin early in the day so that you do not end up working in the dark. Begin near the garage door and work toward your home.

The first step in organizing your garage is to remove every item and place it on the lawn or sidewalk. Ideally, you'll enlist the help of your family for this task, as it can be quite daunting. It can, however, be tackled alone as well; just be sure to bring a cordless radio and to pick a nice day for working so that the work becomes a bit more pleasant.

As you place items on the lawn, separate them into piles by category. Be sure to create two additional piles, one for "throw away" and the other for "give away." When you come across items that have been destroyed because of the elements—moldy furniture, for example, or rusty tools or soggy books—don't deliberate. Just toss them into the garbage. Your work will go faster if you can eliminate as much clutter as possible up-front.

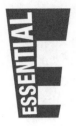

Because the garage can be overwhelming, it can be tempting to get angry at yourself or others when the project goes awry. Keep the words of Julie Morgenstern, professional organizer, in mind: "Go easy on yourself and others when trying to organize these difficult spaces. Everyone in the family is learning a valuable new skill, and it takes time."

Although it is usually best to wait to purchase storage until you know exactly what you'll need, you might be wise to purchase at least a few inexpensive plastic bins (or even garbage cans) to store your items in while you're sorting. Depending on the scope of your garage, cleaning it out could take a few days at least, so you'd be wise to invest in a little portable storage to make things easier as you work. These bins might ultimately become a useful component of your overall storage scheme.

A Good Cleaning

After you've had a chance to pull all of the items out of your garage, you'll want to sweep out your garage and give it a good cleaning. Pull down cobwebs, wash windows, and possibly even hose down the floor. Do whatever it takes to make you feel good about your garage. If you'll be parking your car there after you've organized your storage, remember that you may start using it several times a day. You don't want to be inhaling dust, bugs, and mold every time you exit and enter your car.

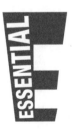

If you must fit two cars into a small garage, try this: Hang two tennis balls from fishing wire, each located to brush the center of your windshield as you pull in. This will help you get each car into the proper spot and prevent you from hitting anything that is stored along the back wall of your garage.

If there are grease spots, you'll want to try to get them up immediately. Concrete floors are porous and the stains can become permanent if you don't tackle them quickly. Although people often neglect the garage floor, spots under your car can provide useful information for troubleshooting problems with your car. If you're leaking oil, you'll want to have your car checked, for example. If you're leaking antifreeze, you'll want to get that leak fixed so that your car doesn't overheat! Consider those spots on the garage floor important tools in diagnosing problems with your car, and try to keep a clean slate so that you can stay on top of potential hazards.

The eHow Web site (www.ehow.com) offers these tips for removing oil stains from your garage or driveway. You may be able to get the oil up with just one or a few of the steps, but if the stain is really bad, you may have to try all of the remedies.

- Pour cola over the oily areas and let it seep overnight. The following morning, lather some dishwashing liquid in a bucket. Rinse the cola with the soapy water and then hose it off.
- Next, add baking soda, cornmeal or sawdust to the oily spots. If you're working with a dry stain, wet it so that you'll have a pasty texture when the absorbent powder is added. Then scrub with a brush or broom.
- Add automatic dishwasher detergent to the spot. You do not need to rise off the baking soda or sawdust. Leave this mixture on the floor for several minutes and then pour boiling water over the area. Scrub with a stiff brush and rinse.
- If none of these simpler remedies work, purchase a commercial concrete cleaner or grease solvent. Carefully follow the instructions on the container.
- Follow each remedy by hosing down the area and letting the area air dry.

To prevent oil spots in the future, you can seal your garage floor. This will make it much easier to keep clean and will prevent future stains. If you choose to paint the floor, the sealant can function as a primer. If you do paint, why not use a bold color that you love? You can afford to take color risks in the garage. Also, by adding a color you enjoy to the garage, you may find that it is easier to keep it clean. Dark, dingy spaces provide little inspiration for the ongoing work of organizing and maintaining a space.

EHow offers the following tips for sealing your garage floor:

- Scrub the floor with a concrete cleaner and degreaser. If the floor has stains, leave the cleaner on for up to 30 minutes before scrubbing. Rinse well.
- When the floor is dry, put the sealer in a paint tray. Use a paint roller to roll the sealer onto the floor. Slowly work your way out of the garage. Though you want to use a generous amount of sealant, make sure that you remove all puddles. Keep in mind that sealant can also leave stains and that you want to keep your garage door open and run a fan for ventilation.
- Do not apply a second coat of sealant, but do wash your tools quickly in a bucket of warm, soapy water.

As you clean out your garage, you'll also want to make sure that your drains are functioning well. You'll want to clean them out by hand in the fall and spring, and you may need to bring in a plumber to unclog them if a problem becomes serious. If your garage is attached to your home, a clog could cause flooding, so you'll want to attend to these drains even when they are just becoming slow, but still function. A slow drain can quickly become a completely clogged drain.

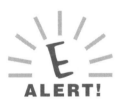
ALERT!

Make sure that all of your garage drains are clear and functioning well. Hosing off the floor will also give you the opportunity to check on the drain efficiency. If they're draining slowly or not at all, you'll want to declog them before you put anything back into your garage.

As you clean your garage and survey the items that have been stored there, take note of any signs of damage done by weather or pests. If there have been pests in your garage, you'll want to greatly reduce the number of items stored in your garage until you're able to identify the problem and solve it. Take note of which items attract pests and which ones suffer damage from the elements, and find a new home for these types of things.

Pest-Proofing Your Garage

You are most likely to encounter evidence of pests in garages that haven't been properly sealed. The garage door is a point of entry for many little critters. The best way to check whether your garage door is sealing properly is to lie on the floor inside and look for light filtering in. Over several years, the rubber seal on the bottom of an automatic garage door does wear out, so you'll want to check the seal periodically.

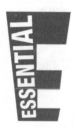

Pay special attention to the corners of the rubber seal on the bottom of your garage door. Be aware that if you have gaps even the size of a sixteenth of an inch, spiders and insects will be able to enter. Pencil-sized gaps (about a quarter-inch tall) will accommodate mice. If you have half-inch gaps, rats can squeeze their way in.

The best way to seal your garage door is to have it fitted with a rubber seal. Keep in mind that these seals do not wear well through the winter and can break down over time, so you may periodically need to replace them. If your garage is connected to your home, make sure that any openings where wires or pipes enter are properly sealed as well. If the cracks are small enough, you can seal them with a caulking gun.

If your garage shows any evidence of weather damage, you'll want to try to identify the source of the problem so that you can reduce expensive structural damage to your garage—a leaky roof, for example, is a problem that will only get worse over the years. Although you probably won't want to tackle these larger issues while you're organizing, make a note on your to-do list to contact a professional mason or roofer as soon as you've gotten your garage put back together.

Storage Solutions

After you've organized your belongings into categories, you'll want to begin to plan storage for the items you'll keep there. Keep your garage empty, and drive your car into it. Then take a piece of chalk and outline your car on the floor. Make sure you open the doors of your car to ensure that you leave ample clearance to get in and out of your vehicle(s). Finally, measure the remaining space to determine which types of storage might work for you.

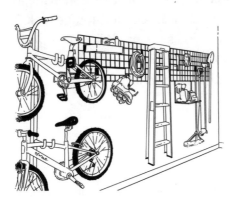

An orderly garage.

Hazards in the Garage

If you do store dangerous tools and chemicals in your garage, you may want to purchase storage that locks to keep children away from these hazards. You'll also want to install both a smoke detector and a carbon-monoxide detector in your garage and check them every six months to ensure they remain operational.

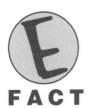

FACT

Work with your children to create a mini parking lot on the garage floor. You can use paint or heavy-duty tape to create "lanes" or "stalls" for these items. Not only will your items have specific homes in the garage, your children will know where they are and be able to put away their own bikes, scooters, and sports equipment.

If you add shelves to your garage, you'll want to keep in mind that items stored on shelves can attract children, so you'll want be careful to prevent little climbers from trying to scale the shelves. You can bolt shelves to the wall, and if you have a large storage component, you can make it extra safe by storing the heaviest things on the bottom and the lighter ones near the top. If you store a ladder in your garage, be sure to hang it horizontally to discourage children from climbing on it.

As you consider the best way to store items in your garage, think in terms of durable, hardy storage solutions, such as metal shelving and bins. For sports items, you might invest in a tension-mount storage rack. This will ease the strain on your bike's tires. If you store garden tools in your garage, you can purchase an upright tool organizer, or mount yard implements (shovels, rakes, and brooms) directly to the wall.

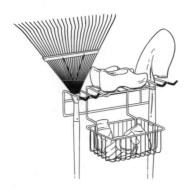

Avoid clutter and find your tools easily by installing wall racks in your garage.

Because you won't spend much time in your garage admiring the aesthetics, focus on function alone when purchasing storage units for your garage. In Appendix A in the back of this book, you'll find more detailed information about how to order storage implements for your garage.

Maintaining Your Car

In the glove compartment of your car, keep a maintenance log of all work that's done on your vehicle. In a file kept at home or in your car, keep copies of all maintenance and repair receipts, warranty information, and other related records. Each time you have work done on your car, ask when the next scheduled maintenance should be done. Mark your calendar or make a notation in your planner or PDA to remind you what needs to be done and when.

Also, try to get all of your car work done at a single location, whether at your local dealership, gas station, or mechanic. This will ensure that you don't overlap maintenance procedures or do maintenance that isn't necessary, such as replacing your car's air filter too often.

While most cars manufactured today are capable of lasting well over 100,000 miles, to keep your car operating smoothly, you'll want to have the items in the following sections checked regularly. Visiting your car's dealership for scheduled maintenance or having the oil changed every 3,000 miles, for example, will help ensure that your car is maintained properly.

Air Filtration

Automobile engines draw air from outside the vehicle to assist in the burning of fuel. About 12,000 gallons of air are needed for every gallon of gasoline used. The vehicle's air filter removes dust, dirt, and other particles from the airflow before it reaches the engine. Air filters become dirty and wear out over time, and should be replaced based on the manufacturer's recommendations or on an inspection during a service. The positive crankcase ventilation (PCV) system draws gasoline fumes out of the engine crankcase and reburns them in the engine. This keeps the engine cleaner and reduces air pollution as well. These fumes pass through the PCV valve on their way to the engine intake manifold. PCV valves become restricted and sometimes clogged with dirt and should be inspected or replaced at regular intervals.

Battery

Don't let the battery stand in a discharged condition. Always keep the acid level between the lower and upper lines marked on the front side of the container. Keep battery tops clean, dry, and free of corrosive matter. Protect the battery from strong impacts or shocks. Clean battery terminals to prevent corrosion. Inspect the vent tube, ensuring that it's not bent, twisted, or clogged.

Brakes

The brakes should never be binding and the car should always be able to roll freely. If your handbreak shows a tendency to stick and cause a drag, mention this at your next service.

Chassis Lubrication

A vehicle's suspension usually consists of numerous moving parts. Heavy grease is injected between the moving joints to prevent wear and metal-to-metal contact. Points that may need greasing include steering components and front-and-rear suspension parts.

Climate Control (Air Conditioning)

Much like your refrigerator at home, an automotive cooling system uses an evaporator, condenser, and compressor to remove heat from the air. Air from the passenger compartment is circulated past the refrigerant-filled evaporator, and then back into the passenger compartment. The refrigerant makes the hot air's moisture condense into drops of water, removing the heat from the air. Periodic service is required to keep the system running at its peak during hot periods.

Engine Lubrication (Oil)

Motor oil is the lifeblood of your car. When the vehicle is running, motor oil circulates through the engine to lubricate the moving parts and reduce friction. It also cools the engine, allowing it to operate at safe temperatures. Quality motor oils contain additives that clean internal engine parts by breaking down contaminants. When the proper viscosity is used, motor oil promotes easy starting at all temperatures. Changing the oil is the best preventive maintenance for an engine. Clean motor oil will prolong the engine life and increase fuel economy. Oil should be replaced following manufacturers' recommendations, which is usually every 3,000 miles for most vehicles.

Fuel Injection

With more efficiency than the older-style carburetor, fuel-injection systems control fuel use and actually spray gasoline into the engine when needed. Using fuel injection, the engine combines gas vapors and air to create a combustible air-fuel mixture. The spark plugs ignite the mixture, creating a series of small explosions that drive the wheels and make the car go. Fuel-injection systems vary the richness of the mixture to suit different operating conditions.

Most automotive experts recommend that fuel-injection systems be professionally cleaned once each year. When possible, use a fuel-additive cleaner every three months.

Lights

Burned-out bulbs should be promptly replaced to keep the vehicle operating in a safe manner. Halogen bulbs that are improperly replaced will have a shorter life and will not illuminate the road as effectively.

Radiator

The radiator system should be serviced according to the manufacturer's recommended mileage interval. This includes a system flush, fluid replacement, and a pressure test of the radiator cap.

Tire Pressure

Tires provide traction for moving a vehicle and assist the brakes in stopping. When properly inflated, they absorb bumps on the road and provide a smooth ride. To operate smoothly, it is essential that a tire and wheel be properly inflated and balanced. Tire imbalance will cause a poor ride, excessive tire wear, and steering and suspension-unit wear (due to continual shaking). To compensate for variations in tire wear, most manufacturers recommend a tire rotation and balance every 6,000 miles.

Transmission

The automatic transmission assumes the task of shifting gears. Most automatic transmissions use a hydraulic system to monitor engine RPMs and select the appropriate gears. Like the engine, fluid circulates through the system to lubricate and cool the moving parts, and a replaceable filter removes impurities. Automatic transmission fluid should be replaced following the manufacturer's recommended mileage interval. Under normal circumstances, the transmission pan gasket and filter should not need to be replaced prior to the 100,000-mile change (assuming that the transmission fluid has been changed following manufacturer's guidelines).

Windshield Wiper Blades

Wiper blades remove rain and snow from the windshield to improve visibility while driving. Over time, hot and cold temperatures and extreme weather conditions cause the wiper materials to break down. Replace them every six months or when visibility is diminished. Each time you get gas, take a moment to wipe off the blades using a rag or paper towel (and if possible, some rubbing alcohol).

Planning for Emergencies

Within your car, you should always keep a first-aid kit and roadside-emergency kit. You will need to customize your roadside kit to make it appropriate for your local climate. Those who live in cold-weather climates, for example, will want to keep items that can be used to stay warm should the car break down, as well as shoveling and deicing implements should the car slide off the road.

Here is a list of items that you might want to keep in your car at all times (allowing for customization for your particular climate):

- Sand or rock salt for traction (in case you get stuck in snow or icy conditions)
- An old scarf and an old belt for emergency hose repairs
- Battery jumper cables (if you can purchase jumper cables that don't require another car, all the better)
- First-aid kit and blanket
- Flashlight with extra batteries, flares, matches
- White cloth to tie to antenna to signal emergency
- Funnel
- Pad and paper
- Plastic jug of water, PowerBars, chocolate, and other nonperishable food items
- Pliers, a wrench, a rubber hammer, a folding shovel, a standard screwdriver, wheel chock, work gloves, fluorescent safety vest, and mechanic's wire

In addition, make sure that your cell phone is always fully charged when you leave your home in your car.

Organization Within Your Car

Even if your car is small, you can find clever spaces to store the items you need on the road. Many car manufacturers offer add-on accessories to make storing and transporting various items easier. Check with your car dealer for a list of accessories available for the make and model of your vehicle.

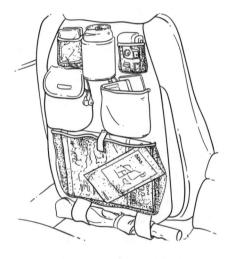

Organize your car.

Some of the most useful organization items you may want to add to your vehicle include a coin sorter (for toll money and parking meters), a holder for sunglasses, a cellular-phone holder/hands-free kit, and a CD holder. You may also want to purchase a plastic container to store car-cleaning products, to be kept in your garage or in your trunk.

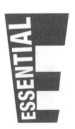

To keep your glove compartment organized, purchase a vinyl portfolio for storing maps and papers (such as your registration and vehicle owner's manual). At least once per month, sort through your glove compartment and throw away garbage and other useless items.

If you have small children, the task of keeping the car clean can be a daunting task. Because you'll often be carrying children, diaper bags, and other items when you exit the car, you can expect to often have a bit of clutter in your car. Go easy on yourself with this—you have a lot to balance! Still, it might be wise to set aside fifteen minutes (ideally, the same time each week) when you're alone to sneak out to the car and clear out old french fries, plastic cups, wrappers and any other items that have accumulated.

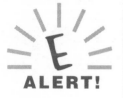

The garage can be a dangerous place for kids, especially if you store chemicals there. Keep all chemicals out of reach or in a locked cabinet, and never let your children play in the garage unattended. Also, have your garage door inspected annually to make sure that it is working properly and will not close on a small child or pet.

As soon as your kids are old enough to help carry items to the house, train them to be your helpers in this task. Also, you may have to vacuum out your car more frequently than your kid-free neighbors. Consider setting aside a regular time each month for car care—if you need to, take it to the gas station and vacuum it out, or delegate this task to your spouse. Although it can be costly, you might also want to have an annual "detail clean." If you can pay somebody else to attend to the deep cleaning, you'll have a far easier time managing the more mundane work of keeping the car orderly. Keep in mind, however, that this detailed cleaning can be expensive. Depending on where you live, it can cost several hundred dollars. Still, some people do feel that the long-term benefits of having the detail clean outweigh the costs.

Rewarding Work

As you begin to get the clutter organized and under control in your garage, you'll begin to experience the benefits. Although you may not often realize how much the clutter kept in your garage drains your energy, when you begin to clear it out, you'll feel as if you have a larger home. Your cars will be happier if they can park there (and so will you, come winter mornings). You'll also save money when your supplies are easy to access because you won't accidentally purchase things you already own. Who knows—by making your garage orderly and finding safer ways to store the dangerous items, you could even save a life. Just as we never really know how much clutter costs us, it is also hard to know, until we begin to tackle it, how much can be gained by bringing order to these often-overlooked spaces.

Chapter 18

Cleaning, Simplified

Cleaning and organizing are closely related. It's difficult to clean until you've reduced your clutter (professional cleaners estimate that purging cuts cleaning time by 40 percent). After you've organized, cleaning brings that final polish to your home. Just as you've struggled to develop organizational strategies that will work over the long haul, you'll also want to develop cleaning strategies that are simple and effective and will work for years to come. This chapter will offer cleaning tips—from speed cleaning to green cleaning and everything in between.

18

Expect Imperfection

Perfectionism can be paralyzing, just as a willingness to embrace imperfection can be liberating. Cleaning is always a work in progress because life is messy—the more people and animals that share a space, the messier it becomes. One of the best ways to adapt yourself to this reality is to expect that you probably won't be able to achieve constant perfection on every front all the time.

Once you've been able to relax into this reality, you'll be better able to develop cleaning systems that will be adaptable to a variety of circumstances. You might want to think in terms of developing weekly (or even daily) rituals. You could either plan to run a load of laundry each day (if your situation warrants that) or you could plan to devote a day each week to the laundry. The FlyLady recommends that certain tasks be delegated to specific days—for example, you could plan to pay bills on Friday, do laundry on Saturday, and reserve vacuuming for Monday. This type of system can keep you from feeling overwhelmed, because you simply focus on the task that you've planned to do on a single day instead of feeling swamped by undone tasks and worrying about how to manage them all. This kind of system might also allow you to keep your home more consistently clean because you'll be rotating through the major weekly tasks instead of procrastinating for weeks on end on the projects that you find least desirable.

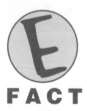

FACT

Mahatma Gandhi was able to embrace his weakness along with his strengths. He wrote, "My imperfections and failures are as much a blessing from God as my successes and my talents and I lay them both at his feet."

Whatever kind of cleaning system you adopt, allow for flexibility. Allow yourself to fail without becoming overly critical. Most people were never really taught to clean well—this is a skill that can be learned with time, patience, and persistence. Different phases of your life will place different demands on you, and sometimes you'll find yourself in a messier home. Just be realistic about what is possible within the confines of your own life, pace yourself, and continue to take steps toward your goals. Know that you'll surely hit obstacles along the way, but if you're not too daunted by imperfection, you'll be able to overcome them. A professional house cleaner offered this advice to Victoria Moran about cleaning: "You have to pretend you're cleaning someone else's house," she said. "Stack anything that hasn't been picked up. Don't read the magazine, answer the letter, or play with the Frisbee. Just stack the stuff and clean." She also said that the key to efficient housekeeping is to do the job "quickly, imperfectly, and without emotional investment."

Speed Cleaning

If you want to dramatically reduce the amount of time you spend cleaning, purchase the book *Speed Cleaning* by Jeff Campbell and the Clean Team. This book will show you how to move from room to room, tackling each part of the room only once. It will help you not only spend less time cleaning, but also to spend less money on cleaning products. You can also learn more about speed cleaning by visiting *www.thecleanteam.com*.

Here is a paraphrase of some of the helpful tips that can be found on the Web site:

- Work around the room one time—and one time only. Carry your equipment with you (in a pocketed apron, for example) so that you don't have to frequently interrupt your work to go searching for supplies.
- Begin at the top and work down. Because gravity pulls dirt and debris downward, it makes no sense to clean the floor before cleaning the counter. If you begin at the top and work down, you'll save precious time and energy.
- Skip clean spots. Don't become so invested in the work of cleaning that you clean surfaces that don't demand it. If you see just a few fingerprints or smudges, just wipe those down and ignore the rest.
- Keep moving. After an area is clean, do not continue to labor there. Your goal is to move as quickly as possible through the house, and lingering will slow you down.

- Use tools that really work. In some cases, you'll need to invest in heavier-duty tools to tackle tougher jobs. Keep all cleaning tools and supplies in good shape so that you won't waste time on leaky bottles, broken brooms, and vacuums that have lost their ability to pick up dirt effectively.
- Make sure you put your tools back in exactly the same spot each time. Otherwise, you'll lose time hunting for them.
- Be attentive to the work at hand and you'll be more successful.
- Pay attention to the amount of time it takes to speed clean your home and strive to get a little faster each time.
- Use both of your hands and you'll dramatically increase your speed. Finish one step with one hand and start the next job with the other.

With cleaning, there are many shortcuts you can take. Be creative about developing your own strategies for making the work fun and efficient. The FlyLady, for example, recommends that you learn to clean the tub while you're in it. She says that you can manage bathtub rings with just a little bit of soap on a washcloth. You might also consider adding baking soda to your bath and wiping the tub down afterward. Baking soda not only relaxes sore joints, but it is also a great, nontoxic, effective cleaner.

Embrace Baking Soda

Baking soda is a cheap, environmentally friendly alternative to harsher cleaners. It is so safe that you can use it on your teeth and in baking, but you can also use it to scour tiles, scrub toilets, remove the grime from sinks, get rid of odors in the refrigerator and on carpets, and wipe down your kitchen counters. This all-purpose household item is a great product to always have on hand.

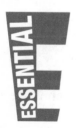

Less junk mail means less clutter, and less clutter means less cleaning. You can reduce the junk mail you receive by sending a request that your name be removed from all mailing lists to: Stop The Mail, P.O. Box 9008, Farmingdale, NY, 11735-9008.

Another way to reduce the amount of time you spend cleaning is to be attentive to dirt before it even enters your home. Purchase a high-quality doormat that is about function rather than aesthetics.

Remove Your Shoes

In many countries around the world, it is standard practice to remove shoes before entering a home, a temple, a church, or a mosque. In these contexts, keeping one's shoes on is considered a sign of great disrespect. In your home, you can reduce the amount of dirt and cleaning by leaving your shoes (and asking guests to leave their shoes) at the front door. Your hard-wood floors and tiles will hold up better without rough shoes to contend with, and much carpet soiling can be avoided. Purchase some slip-on shoes for outdoor use (such as clogs or sandals) so that you can quickly slip your shoes off and on in a pinch.

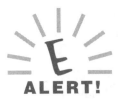

ALERT!

According to professional cleaners, as much as 85 percent of the dirt in your home comes from outside and has made its way in on the bottom of your shoes or in the paws of your pets. You can reduce exposure to lead dust by almost 60 percent if you wipe your shoes on a sturdy mat and leave them outdoors.

Not only is it practical from a cleaning perspective to keep one's shoes at the door, the dirt that comes into your home may actually pose a safety hazard. According to the Environmental Protection Agency (EPA), you can reduce exposure to lead dust by leaving your shoes outside. A report called the "Door Mat Study" presents the theory that soil that has been contaminated by lead causes almost all of the lead contamination inside your home. If you consistently leave your shoes outdoors, you may also be able to reduce your exposure to pesticides (from the lawn and garden), as well as industrial toxins, allergens, and dust mites.

If it feels inhospitable to you to ask guests to remove their shoes, keep in mind the Japanese custom of supplying guests with slippers to wear. The Japanese actually provide slippers at the door of the home, as well as separate slippers for use in the bathroom. Invest in slippers that are comfortable and aesthetically appealing, both for your own family and for your guests, and you'll likely have no trouble convincing them to leave their shoes at the door.

You might want to also supply guests with a visual cue—in some cases, a shoe rack beside the door will be enough to cue them to your custom of going shoeless indoors. In other situations, you might need to create a sign and hang it on your door, as Americans are not generally accustomed to removing their shoes every time they enter a home. Most guests will respect your policy, even if it feels a little awkward to you to ask them to remove their shoes.

Messy Pets

If you have pets, you know that as much as they enrich your life, they also generate a good deal of fur and soiling that must be dealt with. If you have a dog that sheds frequently, you can spend less time picking up hair if you devote just a few minutes each day to brushing the dog. Not only do most dogs relish the attention, but brushing the dog can be relaxing for the dog owner. Instead of being forced to pick up hair all over the house, most hair will be consolidated on the dog brush and can be immediately transferred to the garbage.

If you have trouble keeping up with cat hair, purchase a Zoom Groom, a rubber, massaging brush that cats love (after they get used to it). The Zoom Groom will quickly and efficiently remove excess hair from your cat so that you will not need to be chasing hairballs all over the house.

You might consider giving your cat hairball-preventive treatments every week or every few days, depending on the length and condition of your cat's hair. This treatment will help prevent vomiting because of hairballs.

Cats also tend to track litter away from their litter box. If this is a problem with your cat, purchase a special mat at a pet-supply store. You might consider storing two litter boxes in the tub (one over the drain). By the time the cat has jumped out of the tub, litter has been shaken from his feet and you can easily sweep it up with a small brush.

Making It Fun

One of the best ways to increase your cleaning efficiency (and your efficiency in almost any area of life) is to find ways to enjoy the task. If you can find ways to transform cleaning from a chore into a game, you're halfway there. One time-tested pick-up game involves choosing a certain number of items, setting a timer, and racing against the clock to get these items picked up.

Race Against the Clock

Many people feel that this kind of game can make cleaning a lot more enjoyable and manageable. If you know you're going to set the timer and only clean for a designated amount of time, you're less likely to feel overwhelmed by the scope of the task. It is always easier to take on a five-minute project than it is to attempt to tackle a two-hour one. Another benefit of transforming cleaning into a game is that it is much easier to get children involved in a fun game or race than it is to try to get them involved in household "work."

Cleaning with Kids

If you're tired of cleaning up after your kids, challenge them to join in. Visit any well-run preschool room and you'll see many ways that teachers integrate the work of cleaning into the school day. In some preschools, children sing a song as they clean. In others, children are just reminded to clean up after themselves after meals and snacks. While kids may balk at these kinds of directives at home, they generally obey their teachers because they understand from the beginning that cleaning is part of the arrangement.

If you want to make clean-up fun for your children, there are a few things to keep in mind. First, just as you need not (and should not) demand perfection from yourself in the domestic realm, don't expect perfection from your kids. Think of every cleaning effort on their part as "training" for them. If you encourage and point out the good work they're doing, they'll be more inclined to keep going. If you criticize and correct, they're likely to become discouraged and quit. Either ignore their failings so that they can develop a long-term positive association with cleaning or offer suggestions in an encouraging way, such as, "You're doing a great job folding the towels. Would you like me to show you how I roll socks?"

You can also get really creative with children and cleaning. Try making sock puppets for dusting and have a contest to see who can pick up the most dirt in a set amount of time. Or put on a CD and every time a song ends, switch to the next chore. Especially in your child's bedroom, allow him to take part in organizing the space in a way that is logical to him. If you always do the organizing for him, you may often find the room in chaos because the child does not understand your system. Help him develop his own kid-friendly systems. It's also a good idea to invest in kid-sized cleaning implements when children are small so that they can mimic you as you sweep, vacuum, and dust. This way, cleaning might feel less intimidating to them as they grow older.

Green Cleaning

Increasingly, people are searching for cleaning methods that are safe, cheap, and efficient. During pregnancy, especially, many women cannot tolerate the smell of many of the more toxic cleaners, such as bleach and oven cleaners. Although limited exposure to household cleaners may not cause harm to human health, nobody knows for sure what the threshold is. At what point do household cleaners become a threat to those who live in a home? Some studies suggest that certain people—such as children and the elderly—are more vulnerable to negative health impacts from household cleaners than are more resilient groups.

An Economical Choice

While organic foods typically cost more than "conventional" foods, this trend generally does not carry over into cleaning products. While purchasing ready-made natural cleaners at a health-food store may be more expensive than purchasing cleaning products at your local drugstore, there are many simple household items that are cheap to stock, easy to work with, and nontoxic. These items, which most people already have on hand, can assist you as you begin to explore green cleaning.

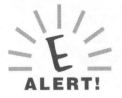

If you use conventional house cleansers, never mix products—especially products containing bleach. Some people have actually died from the fumes created by their accidental toxic blends. Also be sure to rinse well between products to prevent them from mingling. Be mindful as well that although baking soda is a gentle and safe cleaner, when it is combined with bleach, it becomes toxic. Never mix bleach with any chemical or "natural" cleaner.

Not only are these items cheaper than conventional household cleaners, it can be fun to "play the chemist" by mixing up your own green cleaners. A small amount of lavender oil or lemon can bring a fresh aroma to many of these cleaners. Experiment with these products until you find combinations that work for your home.

Here is a list of Green-Cleaning Products, as well as possible uses for each of them. This list comes from Robyn Griggs Lawrence's book *The Wabi-Sabi House: The Japanese Art of Imperfect Beauty*:

- **Olive oil:** Mix 3 parts oil to 1 part vinegar for a clean shine on your wooden furniture
- **Club soda:** Can be used to clean windows and give fixtures a shiny gleam
- **Vinegar:** Ideal for cleaning hardwood floors, and can be used to wipe down grease, diminish soap buildup, and deodorize
- **Borax:** Can kill mold and disinfect
- **Salt:** When mixed with water, this combination can kill bacteria
- **Baking soda:** Can be used to scour and remove odors, and can be combined with vinegar to clean stainless steel

If you clean the inside of your home with nontoxic products, you and your family might become healthier as well. The U.S. Environmental Protection Agency has determined that in many homes, levels of indoor pollution can be somewhere between two to five times higher than outdoor pollutants. Surprisingly, newer homes (those built after 1970) are at a greater risk for this problem because these homes tend to be better sealed against the elements than older homes. While these homes are generally more heat-efficient than their older counterparts, the tight seal on the windows and doors also prevents household toxins—not just those from cleansers, but also carbon monoxide from gas appliances—from escaping. According to an article called "Healthier Indoor Air" by Aisha Ikramuddin in *The Green Guide #76*, well-sealed homes also give rise to dust mites and mold. "Whenever possible, ventilate," she writes. "Let your home breathe and you'll breathe better."

Do You Need a Hand?

As you become more realistic with yourself about your skills and capacities, consider hiring a cleaning person. This hiring does not have to be a substantial investment. You could hire a cleaning person to come just once a month, for example, or every other week. Even if you are on a tight budget, a cleaning person might still be in your budget if you can find ways to reduce your overall spending.

The cost of hiring a professional cleaning person varies a great deal depending on where you live. In a rural area, where the cost of living is generally lower than a larger city, you can expect to pay less than in a major urban area.

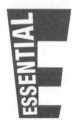

Victoria Moran on hiring a cleaning person: "Getting this kind of help is not self-indulgence. It is time management . . . I look at having her clean my house the way I look at having the dentist clean my teeth: I do the daily stuff; she does the deep cleaning."

Although everyone can develop cleaning skills and routines that work for them, certain situations may make hiring a cleaning person particularly useful. If you work from home, for example, you'll probably want your environment to be reasonably tidy. This will help you to better function as a professional. If you consistently struggle to balance your desire for a clean home with your work deadlines, you might hire somebody to help with the cleaning details. This person can tackle the weightier chores such as mopping and scrubbing out the tub, while you and your family work together to manage the lighter daily maintenance work.

Although cleaning is often thought of as a chore, it can be simplified, and in some cases even enjoyed, if you find a deeper meaning in the work. The more you strategize about cleaning solutions that will work for you, the more likely you are to feel involved in and challenged by the process. Cleaning does not just have to be about the final product, but the actual process can be good for you—cleansing your mind and giving you a break from the more abstract work that might be associated with your job. As Victoria Moran writes, "In the everyday maintenance of our homes, we have the option of experiencing peace, contentment, and that safe feeling of being part of something that is large and grand and good."

Chapter 19

Planning a Move

Along with the loss of a loved one and divorce, moving is one of life's most stressful experiences. But moving does not have to feel like a crisis. If you break your move into small steps, it will become more manageable, and you can keep your serenity even in the midst of all those boxes. This chapter will bring some method to the madness that so often characterizes moves.

Don't Panic

Moving can feel like an insurmountable job. For many people, the task feels so daunting that they are tempted to put it off to the last possible moment, and then it really does feel like a disaster. Instead of trying to avoid all thoughts of the move, begin making lists early on (you'll be glad for those lists when the chaos starts to mount). You can chart out your course of action by creating a "moving schedule," and thus, begin to take small, concrete steps toward moving.

The Clutter Crunch

While you may have wanted to get the clutter in your home under control for some time now, moving might just give you that final push to really crack down on clutter. If you're not sure you're going to move but you're beginning to entertain it as a possibility, the best thing you can do is purge. If you do move, purging will make the move more manageable, and if you don't move, purging will make your home nicer anyway (so you might even lose the desire to move). Purging is a win-win situation.

One way to get aggressive about clutter is to rent a dumpster. While this may seem drastic, you need to think in terms of just getting as much stuff out of your home as possible. A dumpster will allow you to move bulk and volume without having to plan in extra time to take frequent trips to the drop-off charity of your choice. Another option, which is free and more convenient, is to call one of these charities and have them come to your home on a weekly basis to pick-up items. If you know that someone is driving to your home to carry off your clutter, the deadline pressure may help you get a good deal done in a small amount of time.

Realtor Missions

Even before you put your home on the market, Marla Cilley, the FlyLady, recommends that you perform "realtor missions" in your own home. What this means is that you'll come into your home through the front door carrying a clipboard. You'll go through every room and make notations of things that you'd like to change. It is okay to dream big here—you can jot down "Replace living-room carpet" even if you know you can't afford to do it. The point is to constructively brainstorm about how you can improve your living space. You want to try to look at your home as objectively as possible—as if you were a total stranger and you'd never before set foot in your home.

You'll also want to take note of any areas that are full of clutter and need to be cleared out. The idea of possibly putting your home on the market involves a total paradigm shift. While you can still entertain houseguests even if your bedroom closet is in chaos, potential buyers have the right to open every closet door and peer inside. If you can tidy up these spaces, they'll be better able to know what they're buying.

From Private to Public

One of the major adjustments involved with putting your home on the market is that quite suddenly your home will go from your own private haven to a relatively public space. You'll be expected to give a copy of your keys to your realtor, for example, and when you're away she might bring potential buyers through at any time. Likewise, you'll be expected to drop everything—actually, pick up everything—on a moment's notice when the realtor calls to announce that she wants to bring somebody through your home.

If you have children or pets, the suddenly public dimension of your home can be especially difficult to manage. Getting the kids and critters out the door on short notice—as well as picking up after everyone—can be quite a challenge. If you have a kind neighbor nearby, you might ask him if you can bring over your children and pets when the realtor calls. If you can drop them there at least thirty minutes in advance, all the better—you'll need all the time you can get to make your home shine.

How to Move

One of the most stressful aspects of a move is that you'll have to make many decisions quickly. One of the biggest decisions you'll have to make is *how* you'll move. There are a variety of moving options available, suitable to every budget and home size.

Full-Service Movers

By far the most costly option is full-service movers. For many people, full-service movers just aren't an option, but for at least a few lucky souls, this kind of moving service can reduce the stress and ease the physical strain of the move.

These services handle just about every aspect of your physical move. This includes packing your furniture and belongings, supplying all packing materials, loading and unloading the boxes, and unpacking on the other side.

Many factors will influence the cost of this type of move, such as the number of laborers required for the job, the size of the truck, the time of year, the distance of the move, and the amount of furniture and belongings you plan to move.

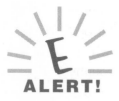

The sooner you decide on your method of moving, the better. As with purchasing airline tickets, you're likely to get a lower bid on renting a truck or hiring full-service movers if you make your reservation well in advance.

If you'll be using a full-service mover, be sure to shop around for the best price. You can visit Web sites such as *www.moving.com* to inquire about available services in your area. Check with family and friends for references—you only want to hire a mover that comes highly recommended to you, as there is a good deal of risk involved with any move. When you have narrowed down your search, you can also check with the Better Business Bureau (*www.bbb.org*) to make sure that the company you want to hire is reputable.

Risks and Benefits

The greatest benefit of full-service movers is that you'll save countless hours packing and moving your furniture. You'll also be spared the difficult decisions of how many boxes to obtain and what size truck to rent. These kinds of questions can be extremely difficult for novice movers to navigate.

There are, however, downsides to full-service movers that you may want to take into account. Aside from the hefty price tag of this kind of move, having other people pack and unpack your belongings can feel like an invasion of privacy. Even if you've invited these people into your home to do just that, come moving day, you might find that you feel uneasy with these strangers handling your possessions. Likewise, some people feel that this kind of move just isn't as satisfying—these people want to set up their own new homes with their own hands. These people feel that the very personal work of settling into a new home should not be outsourced.

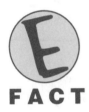

FACT

Full-service movers are registered and/or licensed by a state's department of transportation (DOT). One way to determine whether the moving company you're about to hire is legitimate is to contact the DOT in your state.

When you make your first contact with a full-service mover, be prepared to answer a series of questions. You'll need to know the exact number of miles between where you are currently living and your new home. You'll also need to be able to describe the bulk and quantity of your furniture. They might ask you to estimate how many books you have, for example. They'll also inquire about hard-to-move objects such as pianos.

A full-service mover will provide you with a free quote or estimate that will fall into one of three categories. Make sure that everything you agree to is in writing and is signed and dated by all concerned parties.

Here is a breakdown of the categories:

- **Binding:** In this situation, the mover provides you with a guaranteed price, within a small percentage of deviation. This price is based on a complete list of items to be moved and the type of service requested. To obtain this quote, a representative from the company will have to come to your home and assess your belongings.
- **Nonbinding or Hourly Rate:** Instead of providing an estimate that will detail the cost of your move, this bid will give you an hourly rate. In this situation, you'll be provided with little more than a detailed price list which will detail fees for the moving company's services. While the rates should be based on the movers' previous experience with moves similar to yours, you won't be able to calculate the cost of your move until the move is complete.
- **Not to Exceed:** When a mover gives you a bid, the actual cost cannot exceed this amount. From the movers' standpoint, this quote is binding. In some cases, the move can actually come in under this amount, and you'll pay the lower fee.

After you've consulted with a variety of moving companies, you'll have an idea of the range of services and costs available. The process of obtaining bids can serve as an interview of sorts—hopefully you'll have an opportunity to meet somebody from each company and assess their professionalism and service orientation. Because hiring a full-service mover is costly no matter whom you hire, don't let cost be the determining factor. Choose a reputable mover that you feel you can trust with your belongings, even if you have to pay slightly more.

Pick-up and Delivery Service/Self-Service Movers

If you can't afford a full-service mover, yet you want to be relieved of the burden of renting and driving a moving truck, this type of service might be for you. After evaluating your needs, this type of service will determine exactly what size moving truck you will need and deliver it to your home, typically about two days prior to your move. Then, it's your responsibility to pack up your belongings and place them in your truck.

After the truck is fully loaded, it's picked up by a professional driver and driven to your new home (or, in some cases, to storage).

The price you pay for this service is based primarily on how much space you fill in the truck (based on the truck's weight), as well as the distance of your move.

For an additional fee, you can often hire movers who will help you move the largest and most cumbersome pieces of furniture and heaviest boxes. They can also help you unload your truck at the end of the move. These laborers are usually paid by the hour. Assuming that they are experienced professionals, they could increase the speed of your move—and save your back—because they'll know how to pack the truck efficiently. This may be an especially good option for a single woman who wants to do much of the move on her own but is unable to manage the bulkier items alone.

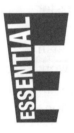

When you reserve your truck, check to see if there are any half-full trucks headed in your general direction. In some cases, you can share a truck with another family for a reduced rate. If you can't fill an entire truck yourself, this option could be very economical for you.

Do-It-Yourself Move

This kind of move entails a few risks, but if you take an organized approach to it, it could be manageable. Keep in mind that although do-it-yourself moves are generally cheaper than other moving methods, these moves are a little harder to budget for because you will incur expenses incrementally. Because most DIY movers are novices, you may find that you actually spend a good deal more than you originally anticipated. Keep in mind that you'll be responsible for fees for: dollies, fuel, furniture pads, hotels, hourly laborers (if necessary), insurance, packing materials (boxes, tape, bubble wrap), tolls, truck-mileage charges, truck-rental charges (including a deposit), as well as possible warehouse and storage fees.

Choosing Packing Materials

If you choose to move on your own, you'll need to obtain packing supplies. Boxes are simple to obtain "on the cheap" from liquor stores, grocery stores, or bookstores. While scrounging for an assortment of boxes can save you some money, it can also cost you in terms of efficiency, because these types of boxes often won't fit together as neatly in your truck as boxes purchased from a professional moving company.

Moving Kits

Inquire about moving kits from these companies, as these kits can contain everything you need to pack up specific rooms of your house or specific belongings. These kits range from starter kits that include several boxes, rolls of tape, bubble wrap, markers, and a utility box, to a protection kit that includes a large variety of bubble wrap, foam cushion, and wraps for dishes and glasses.

When you purchase tape, try to purchase a good amount—more than you think you'll need. You don't want to have to break the flow of your work because you run out of supplies and have to rush to the store. Also, with tape it pays to purchase the clear "tear-by-hand" type. That way, you don't need to waste time losing, recovering, and losing your scissors.

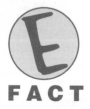

FACT

One way to increase your efficiency is to purchase an apron with large pockets or a front pack. You can store tape, scissors, and colored markers in your pockets, and you'll be less likely to lose them amidst the half-packed boxes.

The FlyLady also recommends that you purchase colored markers and ribbons. This way, you can color-code your boxes, as well as write the room where they are supposed to end up on the exterior of the box. If your boxes are color-coded, you'll be able to immediately identify where each box goes. The more quickly you can sort these boxes into rooms, the less overwhelming the task will feel.

You'll also need garbage bags. If possible, purchase sturdy clear ones so that you don't have to break them open to see the contents. Color-coded ribbons can also increase the efficiency of your move.

The Newspaper Question

Although most people do use newspaper when they pack—it is cheap and readily available—newspaper can be a hassle because it will leave an inky residue all over your hands and belongings. Newspaper is also dusty and dirty. If newspapers are torn, the small fragments can get into the air and irritate your eyes and throat. If possible, purchase plain newsprint instead. The last thing you need after a long day of moving is filthy hands, inky fingerprints on the new white walls, and black streaks on your fine china.

The Moving Schedule

Sometimes the thought of moving can be so overwhelming that it causes an almost total paralysis. You want to get started, but the daunting work ahead can cause you to drag your feet a bit. Instead of thinking in terms of "Moving Day," think in terms of "Moving Months."

You'll want to begin to prepare for your move months in advance. A well-planned move will save you money, spare your health, and decrease your stress. If you move as a family, you'll especially want to take the move in a series of small steps, because your move could be complicated by your children's needs or sudden bouts with the flu or colds.

As soon as you begin to think about moving, you'll want to plan a moving schedule. Use a calendar or planner to determine what needs to be done, and then pencil your tasks into the planner. If you do not always meet your goals on time, do not beat yourself up. Just use your planner as a rough guide for the month ahead. Expect that you'll occasionally be deterred and that you can recover from distractions.

Keep these questions in mind as you plan your move:

- How much time between today and moving day can you dedicate to the move?
- How much time (if any) can you take off from work for move-related tasks?
- Are there any holidays coming up that will allow you extra time to move?
- Are there any tasks that you can complete during your weekly working hours?
- Which tasks are best reserved for the weekends and evenings?
- What time of day are you most likely to be able to tackle moving-related tasks?
- Who will be able to assist you with the details of your move? Might you be able to hire an off-site babysitter or petsitter for the most intense days of the move?
- What is your total moving budget? What steps can you take to keep your move within those confines? Don't forget to plan a cushion for the other side as well—you'll probably have to spend some money on surprise maintenance issues. You may, for instance, need to contact an electrician early on, strip and refinish the floors before you move in, purchase curtains, or replace furniture that does not work in the new space.
- Are there any large pieces of furniture that you'll want to get rid of? Can you place an ad in a local paper or online (try *www.craigslist .org* or *www.ebay.com*) so that you can quickly get rid of some of these larger pieces? Might you be able to make some money from the sale of some of your furniture or possessions that can help you with your move? Keep in mind that people often overvalue their own possessions—you may need to price items drastically lower than what you purchased them for if you want to sell them.

One Move, Week by Week

Here is one possible template for a moving schedule. You can adjust this schedule to make it work for your own needs and circumstances. Although this schedule does not specify weekly goals related to specific rooms of the house, it may be helpful for you to plan to pack up one room a week and to specify your choice of room on the schedule. If you pack just one room at a time, you'll feel less overwhelmed than if you have half-packed boxes all over the house.

Eight Weeks (at Least) Prior to Move

Speak with friends and families about their moving experiences. Begin to research the companies that look most promising and narrow down your options. Contact these companies to obtain bids. If the fee range varies greatly from company to company for similar services, inquire about these discrepancies. Calculate potential moving expenses—contact your employer and the IRS to check on possible assistance and deductions. Create a detailed schedule for your move. Contact a charity to see if they might be willing to do weekly pick-ups, or rent a dumpster so that you can simplify the process by clearing out excess clutter.

Seven Weeks Prior to Move

Create an inventory of all that you own. From this inventory, decide which items you'll move on your own and which you'll need assistance with. Consider placing ads on craigslist.org or eBay for items you don't want to take with you. If you have enough items that a garage sale would be feasible (and if your schedule allows), have one now. Contact your insurance companies to obtain insurance for your move and for your new residence. Begin dealing with change-of-address issues with utilities, credit card companies, and magazine subscriptions. Arrange for a transfer of medical and dental records to your child's new school. Make sure that you obtain your own copies of all medical (especially vaccination) and dental records which can transfer to your new doctors and dentists in your new location. Obtain packing/shipping supplies.

Six Weeks Prior to Move

Begin packing nonessential items. Confirm moving dates with the company you've selected and complete all related paper work. Contact your current landlord and neighbors to discuss your departure. If you will be flying to your new city, purchase airline tickets.

Five Weeks Prior to Move

Cancel local deliveries, such as newspapers, milk, and so on. Continue to pack nonessential items. Order your financial records and paperwork (you may want to purchase a portable, plastic filing box so that you can keep essential records close at hand). Send an e-mail to family and friends with information about your new address.

Four Weeks Prior to Move

Complete change-of-address forms with the post office and IRS. Notify your insurance companies and utility companies of your move. Continue to purge and pack.

Three Weeks Prior to Move

Arrange for a babysitter to watch your kids on moving day. Continue sorting and packing. Return all library books, videos, and items belonging to friends and neighbors.

Two Weeks Prior to Move

Contact utility companies for your new location and arrange for service. Continue to pack. Transfer your finances and bank accounts to branches near your new home. Transfer prescriptions to new pharmacies or inquire about your ability to pick-up prescriptions from a pharmacy in your new town if your prescription is held at a chain pharmacy.

If you are able to hire professional cleaners to clean your home, schedule a cleaning for the day after you move out. This may be a great way to save time—expect that you won't have a lot of extra energy surrounding your old home, but that the new owners will certainly appreciate a professional cleaning job prior to moving in.

One Week Prior to Move

Finish packing. Reconfirm date with your moving company. Pack personal belongings that will travel with you. Empty and defrost your refrigerator. Pack your personal items to travel with you. If you are moving any appliances, prepare them for transfer. Review all paperwork related to your move. Begin packing your unload-first box (this should include essential items such as your toiletries, bedding, towels, paper ware for the kitchen, light bulbs, tools, a flashlight, a notepad and pen for making lists, and possibly your coffee pot and some coffee).

Moving Day

Pack up your bed and last-minute items. Finish packing your "unload-first" box.

Confirm delivery time with movers. During your move, try to be considerate of your neighbors. Try to avoid making too much noise early in the morning or late at night.

Move-In Day

Arrive at your new home before the moving company. Ideally, you will have access to the home at least a few days before the moving company comes so that you can do any last-minute cleaning and preparations. On that first day, if you've moved appliances, make sure they've been properly hooked up and are working properly. Have payment ready for the movers—in most cases they will prefer cash. Check with them in advance, because the last thing you need on your moving day is to have to rush to the bank for cash!

Have a tool kit on hand to fix and assemble furniture. Assemble the beds so that you can sleep in your new home on that very first night. Head to the local grocery store and stock your kitchen with quick snacks that won't make a mess—fruit, PowerBars, fresh bread, milk, nuts, bottled water—anything that will make you feel a little more settled in your new home and keep your blood sugar stable for the work ahead.

Waking Up in Your New Home

That first morning in your new home may be very unsettling. You may feel excited and overwhelmed in turns—relieved that you've made it into your new home with all of your possessions intact yet distressed at all the work that lies ahead. No matter how carefully you've planned your move, your house is likely to feel chaotic on that very first morning.

Pace Yourself

That first morning, treat yourself to the luxury of your regular routines. Perhaps you always drink coffee in the morning—brew yourself a pot and then sit down with a steaming cup and notepad. You can make a list of the work ahead. Often, it is easiest (and least overwhelming) to unpack one room at a time. On your list, note which room(s) you want to tackle first.

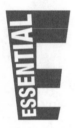

Each time you open a box, plan to unpack it completely, break it down, and take it out to recycling or storage. This will cut down on the chaos. There are few things as confusing as trying to decide what to do next when you're surrounded by two dozen open boxes.

As you begin the work of unpacking, be patient with yourself! Unpacking can take as long as (or longer than) packing because it involves difficult decisions. Don't rush to hang your pictures, either. You can give yourself time to think about where they should go—it doesn't matter if it takes several months. Those blank walls are full of possibilities, symbolic of the infinite possibilities related to your home. Let yourself live with these possibilities instead of forcing decisions before you're ready.

Allow yourself time to settle into your new home, and take frequent breaks so that you don't become overwhelmed.

Create a Quiet Corner

Even if your new home is beautiful, it will probably feel chaotic those first few days as you struggle to bring order to the situation. It would help to create a calm corner where you can rest and recharge. Ideally, this space will include a comfortable chair, a small table for drinks and paperwork, and a lamp so that you're not forced to sit beneath the unfriendly glare of an overhead light.

If you have items of religious or personal significance, place them in your quiet corner so that the space will invite prayers and meditation. As you slowly settle into your new home, this corner can be your refuge. You can return to it again and again to rest and recharge. It can be a place of nourishment, reflection, and peace. A calm zone in the midst of the chaos can help you feel anchored as you begin to settle into your new home. You can reflect the peace you experience there to your family members, and they will feel calmer as a result. And remember, if you continue to take small steps each day to order your home and to make it beautiful, that little corner of peace can grow until it permeates the entire house.

Chapter 20

Bringing It all Together

As you've worked through the chapters of this book, you've hopefully learned a great deal about what works for you in terms of organization. This final chapter will bring together some of the principles outlined in the book, as well as offer ideas about learning to manage the final frontier—your time.

The End of Yo-Yo Organizing

In Julie Morgenstern's book *Organizing from the Inside Out*, she coins the term "yo-yo organizing." This concept is similar to the yo-yo diet habit, where you try one diet after another, often with some temporary success, only to fail in the end. Just as yo-yo dieters often gain more weight than they lose, yo-yo organizers often tackle the clutter in their homes with zeal, only to eventually end up with more chaos and clutter than they began with.

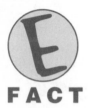

FACT

The ideal solutions are those that wear well with time because they are realistic, are a good fit for your own preferences, personality, and lifestyle, and are flexible enough that they can be modified for each phase of life.

What goes wrong? Why do so many diets (and home-organization methods) fail? According to Morgenstern, the problem is that most of the books and methods focus on external solutions to problems that can only be solved internally. You cannot buy your way out of the chaos—organizational systems work only to the extent that the person who is using them has taken a customized approach to their unique situation, abilities, and personality.

Organizing Your Time

You might find that as you bring order to the different rooms in your home, you become aware of the less-tangible elements of your life—such as time management—that continue to be somewhat chaotic. It might be helpful to think of time as Julie Morgenstern does—in a very concrete way. Just as it is possible to tackle the chaos in your closets, it is equally possible to bring order to the hours of your day.

For Julie Morganstern, time was the last thing she learned to organize. For her, the first steps were bringing order to her home, her purse, her office. Only after she found a way to manage the concrete details of these areas did she find the impetus to learn to organize her time. It was nothing short of a revelation for her to discover that organizing her time was just like organizing her closet. Her overstuffed closets were, in reality, finite spaces that could only contain a finite amount of clothing.

The first step was recognizing that time—although it might feel somewhat abstract in comparison to one's closet—is actually limited. Julie had packed her life so full that it was difficult to see what was important and to prioritize. It is hard to be efficient when you cannot see clearly the items or opportunities before you. Like her closets, Julie needed to peer at her life with open eyes and begin to reconsider the way she spent her time.

Learn to Say No

Just as managing and purging clutter is an essential first step as you seek to bring order to your home, learning to say "no" is an equally essential skill as you seek to organize your time. It is the fastest, most efficient way to declutter your day and reclaim your life. For some people, saying no can be difficult, but as you do it more and more, you experience the rewards—the gift of a streamlined, focused, and productive life—and saying no becomes as much of a healthy habit as the other ones mentioned in this book.

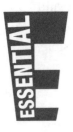

If you want to say no to something but fear you lack the courage, consider the possibility that the chaos in your home might be a direct result of an inability to say no. Sometimes people become so engaged with solving other people's problems that they neglect their own. This kind of neglect often shows up in chaotic homes.

Just as Julie Morgenstern does not recommend that you charge into your cluttered basement or attic without a plan, it might also be helpful to think of time in similar terms. As you struggle to divide your time between jobs, opportunities, and relationships, you might consider creating a criterion for weighing each option.

Sometimes, it can be helpful to consider whether a potential opportunity causes you more exhaustion or exhilaration than it's worth. Although a certain amount of exhaustion is inevitable, if you can say no to more of the opportunities that exhaust you and yes to more of the ones that exhilarate you, you will be happier and more productive.

Long-Term Goals

Another time-management essential is balancing your time between immediate concerns and long-term goals. In many situations, it can be tempting to constantly live as if you're putting out fires—just managing one urgent problem after another. But if you can begin to schedule time into your week to manage situations that are not yet pressing but will become increasingly urgent if ignored, you will simplify your life and gain greater peace of mind.

Every Morning, Create a Detailed To-Do List

You may find it helpful to sit down each morning with a notepad and pen and create a to-do list. This way you'll go into the day with a sense of purpose and priorities. Your list might include your personal and work-related objectives for the day. Or your list may include errands, meetings, appointments, phone calls to make, and e-mails to write. It should also include tasks that bring you closer to achieving your personal, professional, and financial long-term goals. After you create your to-do list, prioritize each task and input the appropriate information into your personal planner, PDA, or other scheduling tool. Ideally, you will plan out as much of your day as possible, leaving a realistic amount of time to deal with unexpected events.

Your to-do list can also keep your household organized and clean. For example, when you're about to embark on a massive clean-up or reorganization project, writing out a to-do list helps you clearly define your objectives, create a time frame, and take a well-thought-out approach to your efforts.

Create a Task List

For the day-to-day tasks that are necessary to run your home and keep it clean, follow these basic steps:

- Create a list of what tasks you need to do (clean the bathroom, do the laundry, change bed linens, vacuum, wash the kitchen floor, go to the dry cleaner, mow the lawn, and so on).

- Determine how often each of these tasks needs to be done.
- Using a calendar, PDA, scheduler, or personal planner, create a schedule for accomplishing these tasks one at a time. For example, cleaning the bathroom may take thirty minutes after work on Mondays. Trips to the dry cleaner can be done on Tuesdays and Thursdays on the way to work or when dropping your kids off at soccer practice.

After you create a to-do list for keeping your home clean and organized, try to work through it one item at a time. Do not become discouraged if you get sidetracked—just pick up where you left off when you have the opportunity.

A Work in Progress

As you begin to better manage your home and time, keep in mind that many things are works in progress. Don't become distressed when things do not go as you'd hoped. As with any major project, there will be setbacks, failures, and unanticipated challenges. If you know that you will hit many bumps along the way, you will be less likely to let them deter you for any length of time.

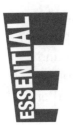

As you develop your methods and slowly become more organized, you'll periodically want to assess your systems and see what is working and what isn't. Sometimes, something that worked well for several months will no longer work well. Be flexible with yourself, and modify your systems (and your goals) depending on the real circumstances you find yourself in.

As you begin to experience the rewards of a more ordered home and schedule, you might find that these aspects of your life become increasingly easy to maintain because they have built-in rewards. It feels good to have a sense of a reasonably ordered life, especially in the face of all of life's uncertainties.

Work Toward Your Goals

As you establish your long-term organizational goals, determine exactly what it will take to achieve each goal. Divide up each long-term goal into a series of short-term or medium-term goals that are more easily achievable. After you create a series of smaller goals, develop a timeline and set specific deadlines. Each time you accomplish one of these smaller goals, you'll be that much closer to achieving one of your long-term goals.

In your mind, you want to know clearly what you're working toward, how much time you have to achieve your objectives, and what possible rewards you can expect upon achieving your goals. You'll want to have a clear sense of why you're working toward a particular objective and what success in that area will mean to you.

Celebrate Success

After you've had an opportunity to develop some organizational skills and habits that work for you, remember to continue to pace yourself. Every domestic success should be celebrated. For most people, taking a few moments to celebrate success can be a helpful way to bring more joy to the work and to ultimately accomplish more.

It can be tempting to become so fixed on your goal that you never take a moment to rest and reflect on all that you've accomplished. Sometimes you might offer yourself incentives such as, "I'll clean out this drawer and then take a break with a cup of coffee," only to find that you get so involved with the work of organizing that you forget about your reward. This kind of approach can cause burnout over the long haul.

Especially when you're faced with a major organizational task, you don't want to have memories of days and days of tackling the clutter in your garage with no break. If the work seems like drudgery, you're likely to procrastinate until it becomes unmanageable. If you take small steps and celebrate each success, you'll have a natural incentive to retain your organizational zeal over the years, when different organizational challenges (a new baby, a move, a death in the family) present themselves to you.

Stay Focused on What Is Real

In Victoria Moran's book *Shelter for the Spirit*, she mentions a friend who, after wiping out her tub, said, "This is the most *real* thing I've done all day." Often, people postpone or dread housework simply because it seems like a waste of time when there are other, seemingly more important, things to do.

The truth is, that the concrete realities of daily life are an essential part of being human, and these simple, manageable tasks, against the backdrop of a seemingly chaotic and unmanageable world, can be comforting to your soul.

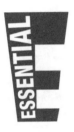

Victoria Moran writes, "In the landscape of our lives, making a home is front and center. The consensus of every major religion—and the majority of people who consider themselves happy—is that the primary tasks of humans is to learn how to love . . . At home, with pretenses hung in the closet next to the business suits, we learn it best."

Take Each Day as It Comes

Knowing that you're returning to an orderly home is a little bit like knowing that you're about to go on vacation—only in this situation, your home becomes your refuge. You don't need to pack and you don't need to spend any money, but you will experience the refreshment and relaxation you need to thrive.

Organizing your home and time are two pieces of the larger project of life—and they will always be works in progress—always involving difficult decisions, and finite resources. The pinch is felt especially when you have small kids at home, pets, and frequent houseguests. All of these little "distractions" are part of the package—because they help you to be more realistic, to realize what is essential. As Lin Yutang said, "Beside the noble art of getting things done, there is the noble art of leaving things undone. The wisdom of life consists in the elimination of nonessentials."

Appendix A

Web Resources

Now that you've developed a plan for organizing your home, you'll want to hone in on the services that will help you to achieve your goals. The following Web resources offer information about specific storage solutions and charitable organizations, as well as contact information for professional organizers.

Organizational Consultants

California Closets
✍ *www.calclosets.com*

Closet Factory
✍ *www.closetfactory.com*

The National Association of Professional Organizers
✍ *www.napo.net*

Organization By Design, Inc.
✍ *www.dressingwell.com*

Storage by Design
✍ *www.storagebydesign.com*

Companies that Carry Organizational Products

The Container Store
✍ *www.containerstore.com*

Container World
✍ *www.storagesources.com*

Frontgate
✍ *www.frontgate.com*

Ikea
✍ *www.ikea-usa.com*

Lillian Vernon
✍ *www.lillianvernon.com*

Organize.com
✍ *www.organize.com*

The Sharper Image
✍ *www.sharperimage.com*

Stacks and Stacks
✍ *www.stacksandstacks.com*

Unique Organizational Products

AeroBed
✍ *www.thinkaero.com*

Brookstone
✍ *www.brookstone.com*

Garage Storage Cabinets
✍ *www.garagestoragecabinets.com*

Restoration Hardware
✍ *www.restorationhardware.com*

Rubbermaid
✍ *www.rubbermaid.com*

Shelving Direct
✍ *www.shelving-direct.com*

Solutions
✍ *www.solutionscatalog.com*

Kitchen/Dining Products, Services, and Information

Kitchens.com
✑ *www.kitchens.com*

Kitchen Source
✑ *www.kitchensource.com*

Kitchenweb
✑ *www.kitchenweb.com*

Set Your Table: Discontinued Tableware Dealers Directory
✑ *www.setyourtable.com*

Williams-Sonoma
✑ *www.williams-sonoma.com*

Landscape and Garage Products and Information

Decks USA
✑ *www.decksusa.com*

Gardener's Supply Company
✑ *www.gardeners.com*

Smith & Hawken
✑ *www.smithandhawken.com*

TIDYGARAGE
✑ *www.tidygarage.com*

Safety Products and Information

Fight Bac!
✑ *www.fightbac.org*

Juvenile Products Manufacturers' Association
✑ *www.jpma.org*

Safe Kids Worldwide
✑ *www.safekids.org*

Safety 1st Childcare Products
✑ *www.safety1st.com*

U.S. Consumer Product Safety Commission
✑ *www.cpsc.gov*

Moving and Storage Resources

AllBoxes Direct
✑ *www.allboxes.com*

American Moving & Storage Association
✑ *www.moving.org*

Extra Space Storage
✑ *www.sus.com*

Hertz Truck & Van Rental
✑ *www.hertztrucks.com*

IRS
✑ *www.irs.gov/formspubs*

LowCostBoxes.com
www.lowcostboxes.com

Moving.com
www.moving.com

Public Storage
www.publicstorage.com

Ryder Truck Rental
www.ryder.com

SelfStorageNet.com
www.selfstoragenet.com

U-Haul
www.uhaul.com

Photo and Scrapbook Resources

AlbumSource.com
www.albumsource.com

Scrapbooking.com
www.scrapbooking.com

Scrapbook-Tips.com
www.scrapbook-tips.com

Charitable Organizations

Careergear.com
✎ *www.careergear.com*

Dress for Success
✎ *www.dressforsuccess.org*

Goodwill Industries International, Inc.
✎ *www.goodwill.org*

The Salvation Army
✎ *www.salvationarmyusa.org*

The Women's Alliance
✎ *www.thewomensalliance.org*

Volunteers of America
✎ *www.voa.org*

Appendix B

Helpful Books

The author wishes to gratefully acknowledge the work of the following authors. These books provided inspiration during the process of writing and researching this book. Should you wish to further explore any of the ideas you've read about in these pages, these resources are a great place to start. They explore a variety of aspects related to homemaking, such as aesthetics, organization, cleaning, and productivity issues.

Allen, David. *Ready for Anything: 52 Productivity Principles for Work and Life* (New York: Viking Penguin, 2003). This book can help you become more efficient, organized, and productive.

Cilley, Marla–The FlyLady. *Sink Reflections* (New York: Bantam Dell, 2002). This extremely down-to-earth and practical book is written in an accessible style and offers many helpful hints for getting your home (and life) in order.

Hollender, Jeffrey et al. *Naturally Clean: The Seventh Generation Guide to Safe & Healthy, Non-Toxic Cleaning* (British Columbia: New Society Publishers, 2006). This book offers an in-depth look at the hazards associated with household cleaners and indoor air pollution.

Lawrence, Robyn Griggs. *The Wabi-Sabi House: The Japanese Art of Imperfect Beauty* (New York: Clarkson Potter, 2004). This book offers an insightful introduction to the concept of wabi-sabi. It is a pleasure to read and is illustrated with beautiful photographs.

Moran, Victoria. *Shelter for the Spirit: Create Your Own Haven in a Hectic World* (New York: HarperCollins, 1998). This book is a personal, reflective guide to creating a home that is both aesthetically pleasing and comforting to your soul.

Morgenstern, Julie. *Organizing from the Inside Out: The Foolproof System for Organizing Your Home, Your Office and Your Life*, 2nd ed. (New York: Henry Holt & Co., 2004). Julie Morgenstern draws from years of experience as a professional organizer, distilling her wisdom into this practical, easy-to-read guide to getting your home in order.

St. James, Elaine. *Simplify Your Life: 100 Ways to Slow Down and Enjoy the Things That Really Matter* (New York: Hyperion, 1994). This quick read offers useful tips for streamlining your home and life, improving your health, and learning to enjoy life's simplest joys.

Index

C